THE EVERYTHING

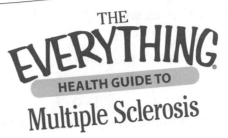

HEALTH GUIDE TO

Multiple Sclerosis

Dear Reader,

There has never been a better time to learn about multiple sclerosis. In your explorations, you're likely to stumble upon great pockets of hope. New diagnostic tools and treatment strategies are part
of the management landscape, and new targets of research come
to the fore each year.

It's important to keep up with these exciting developments
while effectively learning to manage MS. Indeed, knowledge and
diligence comprise the foundation of self-care.

The complexities of MS require those who live with it to be
educated, proactive, and unyielding. Understanding its symptoms,
patterns, and treatments will enable you to take control of your
health and manage your MS effectively. Emotional well-being plays
a big role, too. While you endeavor to stay one step ahead of your
symptoms, you must also create a space where MS comes last in
line. Finding ways to balance the needs of a chronic illness with
your desire to live a full and robust life is one of the most important
things you can do.

We hear so much these days about "empowerment." And while
empowerment is not a cure, we hope the tools set forth in this book
will enable you to be as healthy and happy as you possibly can.
Combined with a sense of hope and optimism, you have every right
to look forward to the future.

Margot Russell

THE

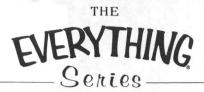

Everything® Health Guides are a part of the bestselling *Everything*® series and cover important health topics like anxiety, postpartum care, and thyroid disease. Packed with the most recent, up-to-date data, *Everything*® Health Guides help you get the right diagnosis, choose the best doctor, and find the treatment options that work for you. With this one comprehensive resource, you and your family members have all the information you need right at your fingertips.

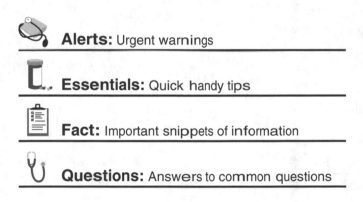

Alerts: Urgent warnings

Essentials: Quick handy tips

Fact: Important snippets of information

Questions: Answers to common questions

When you're done reading, you can finally say you know **EVERYTHING**®!

PUBLISHER Karen Cooper

DIRECTOR OF ACQUISITIONS AND INNOVATION Paula Munier

MANAGING EDITOR, EVERYTHING SERIES Lisa Laing

COPY CHIEF Casey Ebert

ACQUISITIONS EDITOR Lisa Laing

DEVELOPMENT EDITOR Brett Palana-Shanahan

EDITORIAL ASSISTANT Hillary Thompson

Visit the entire Everything® series at *www.everything.com*

THE
EVERYTHING®
HEALTH GUIDE TO
MULTIPLE SCLEROSIS

An authoritative guide to help
you understand symptoms, decide on
treatment, and enhance your well-being

Margot Russell

with Allen C. Bowling, M.D., Ph.D.

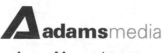

Avon, Massachusetts

For the people across the world who live with multiple sclerosis.
Your courage never fails to inspire me.

• • •

An Everything® Series Book.
Everything® and everything.com® are registered
trademarks of F+W Media, Inc.

Published by Adams Media, a division of F+W Media, Inc.
57 Littlefield Street, Avon, MA 02322 U.S.A.
www.adamsmedia.com

ISBN 10: 1-59869-805-2
ISBN 13: 978-1-59869-805-3

Printed in Canada.

J I H G F E D C B

Library of Congress Cataloging-in-Publication Data
is available from the publisher.

This publication is designed to provide accurate and authoritative information
with regard to the subject matter covered. It is sold with the understanding that
the publisher is not engaged in rendering legal, accounting, or other professional advice. If legal advice or other expert assistance is required, the services
of a competent professional person should be sought.
　　—From a *Declaration of Principles* jointly adopted by a Committee of the
American Bar Association and a Committee of Publishers and Associations

Many of the designations used by manufacturers and sellers to distinguish their
products are claimed as trademarks. Where those designations appear in this
book and Adams Media was aware of a trademark claim, the designations have
been printed with initial capital letters.

The Everything® Health Guide to Multiple Sclerosis is intended as a reference
volume only, not as a medical manual. In light of the complex, individual,
and specific nature of health problems, this book is not intended to replace
professional medical advice. The ideas, procedures, and suggestions in this
book are intended to supplement, not replace, the advice of a trained medical
professional. Consult your physician before adopting the suggestions in this
book, as well as about any condition that may require diagnosis or medical
attention. The author and publisher disclaim any liability arising directly or
indirectly from the use of this book.

This book is available at quantity discounts for bulk purchases.
For information, please call 1-800-289-0963.

All the examples and dialogues used in this book are fictional and have
been created by the author to illustrate medical situations.

Contents

Acknowledgments

I'd like to thank my editor, Lisa Laing, who showed great patience while I researched and wrote about the complex subject of multiple sclerosis. Dr. Allen Bowling was a valuable collaborator and is an important voice in the MS community. Without him this book would not have been possible. I would also like to acknowledge the tireless work of researchers and other foot soldiers in the medical field who endeavor to shine light on the causes and treatment of MS. Finally, I'd like to thank my family—Bill, Kerry, Colleen, and Maggie—for their patience and support. And to Jane, Katherine, and Michele, who continue to inspire me.

Introduction

If you've just been diagnosed with multiple sclerosis, you're likely to feel overwhelmed. Even answering the question "What is MS?" takes a rudimentary understanding of both the immune and central nervous systems. Words such as "T cells" and "demyelinate" require a medical dictionary, so you've barely digested the news before you're confronted with a new vocabulary. And just as you're getting good at understanding what you've got, you're confronted with a whole array of choices for treatment and symptom management.

The truth is that learning to understand and live with MS is a process. And it's a lifelong process, best taken one step at a time. You start out by finding a way to accept your diagnosis, move into education, and then master learning to manage the disease. This doesn't happen in a month or a year, but in a time frame that is uniquely suited to your own way of doing things. And while treatment is best started early, you can ease into other things, such as an exercise routine, a better diet, or joining a support group.

Your MS education will likely come from a variety of places, including your neurologist, local or national organizations, the Internet, books, and pamphlets. But the most important things you'll learn are those things you gain through experience—by living with MS. You get to know your quirks, your temperament, and your limits by living day to day with them. No two people have MS in exactly the same way, so self-knowledge is your most important ally.

Along with understanding the ABCs of this complex disease, you'll also learn something about who you are as a person. This is the unintended but unavoidable consequence of living with chronic illness. You'll find unexpected stores of courage, determination, and hope inside yourself. You'll become familiar with your own limits and frustrations, and in the interim find new ways to do old things. What you may perceive as a future of limits is really just an invitation to define yourself in a new way.

It's the good news about MS that has people talking: the new disease-modifying drugs, the diagnostic tools, and the accelerated race for a cure. There is more reason to be hopeful about MS than ever before, and this new optimism pervades the MS landscape. As the mysteries behind MS slowly come to light, your choices have broadened. These days, there are a variety of drugs to choose from that may alter the course of MS along with its symptoms. There are clinical trials to consider, and alternative therapies—such as yoga—to explore. There are also a multitude of ways to get involved in the cause.

This book is intended to be a helping hand in coming to terms with MS. Not only will it help you to define MS, it will also assist you in learning how to manage MS. Management involves taking good care of your health, creating a network of supportive friends and family, and getting a firm grip on your emotional health. You'll also get a better handle on treatment strategies and learn the best way to control your symptoms.

A diagnosis of MS is often an unwanted guest in your life. It changes the way you see tomorrow and the day after that. But breaking down the tasks in front of you can make it seem less daunting. Knowing that a lot of other people are walking in the same shoes and are living successful and fulfilling lives can ease your sense of isolation.

You've got options. It's what you choose to do that matters.

CHAPTER 1

MS: The Nuts and Bolts

IF YOU'VE PICKED up this book, it is most likely because you—or someone you love—has been diagnosed with multiple sclerosis (MS), or perhaps your doctor has mentioned MS as a possibility. Whatever the case, you may have already discovered that putting MS into perspective can be a challenging process. MS is a complex disease, and one that is especially hard to diagnose. Its symptoms vary widely from person to person, and although researchers have made great strides in understanding the condition, the cause remains a mystery.

What Is MS?

While most everyone has heard of MS, you certainly wouldn't be the first person to lack a full understanding of its nuts and bolts. When MS is suspected or diagnosed, it is not uncommon for someone to ask "What exactly is MS?"

MS is defined as a chronic, inflammatory, demyelinating disease that affects the central nervous system (CNS). What that means in a nutshell is this: MS is thought to be an autoimmune disease that affects the command center of your body's functions—your CNS—resulting in a myriad of neurological symptoms. To get a better handle on the mechanics of MS, you must first understand the roles the CNS and the immune system play.

The Nervous System

The nervous system is composed of two parts:

- The central nervous system is made up of the brain, spinal cord, and optic nerves. It interprets sensory information and sends commands to the muscles.
- The peripheral nervous system (PNS) connects the CNS to the glands, sensory organs, and muscles through a branching network of nerves.

Both the CNS and the PNS are made up of nerves that act as the body's messenger system. Each nerve is covered by a fatty substance called myelin, which provides insulation and helps in the transmission of nerve impulses, or messages between the brain and other parts of the body. MS is exclusive—its sole target is the CNS.

The Role of the Immune System

The immune system is a complex system of cells, tissues, and organs that work together to protect your body from foreign invaders—mostly germs that can cause infection. Although people barely take notice of their immune system, it is incredibly competent, able to recognize millions of enemies, target them, and wipe them out. This is known as an immune response.

Because a healthy immune system has the remarkable ability to distinguish between your own cells and foreign cells, your defense system and your own cells coexist quite peacefully. In abnormal situations, however, the immune system mistakes your own cells for foreign invaders and then launches an attack on the healthy cells and tissues. This is called an *autoimmune response*. A disease that results from this type of faulty immune response is called an *autoimmune disease*. A great number of diseases are believed to be autoimmune in nature, including type-1 diabetes and rheumatoid arthritis. MS is also thought to be an autoimmune disease.

Fact

There are more than eighty known autoimmune diseases affecting approximately fifty million Americans, or one in five people. Of that group, 78 percent are women. Autoimmune diseases are the third most common category of disease in the United States after cancer and heart disease.

Although science is not sure why, it appears that in MS, the immune system has lost the ability to distinguish the good cells from the bad cells and, through the process of inflammation, begins to attack the myelin sheath that coats and protects the nerves. The myelin coating is distributed along the axons of the nerves, the long extensions that carry electric impulses. As the myelin is stripped and destroyed, bare spots or scars (also called *sclerosis*) appear along the nerve in multiple areas—thus the name MS. As a result, signals transmitted from nerve cell to nerve cell throughout the CNS are disrupted or slowed down. Experts once believed that axons themselves were spared during the disease process, but research has shown that the axons can be damaged or broken. Your symptoms depend on the extent of myelin or axon damage and where the damage is located in your CNS. For example, if the myelin sheath along your optic nerve (which connects the eye to the brain) has been damaged, you may have a problem with your eyesight.

Understanding Plaques

Plaques (or areas of scarring) are the hallmark signs of MS, and they can occur at any site where there are myelinated axons within the

CNS. These axons conduct impulses at a very high rate and allow the transfer of information between neurons to facilitate motor function and sensory perception. The location and number of lesions vary greatly from person to person.

Scientists have discovered that the nerves actually try to remyelinate—to restore the insulating myelin along the damaged nerve—but the results are less than perfect. In time, scar tissue builds up and, along with the damaged axons, the ability of the nerve to transmit nerve impulses is compromised or destroyed. Keep in mind that damage to the CNS doesn't happen all at once, but usually occurs in distinct but unpredictable episodes, also known as an MS relapses, attacks, flares, or exacerbations. Relapses are chracterized by the sudden appearance or worsening of a symptom (or symptoms) that lasts at least twenty-four hours. These episodes are usually followed by periods of recovery or remission.

The Role of the Blood-Brain Barrier

And just when you think you've finally grasped it all, the blood-brain barrier comes into play. In simple terms, the blood-brain barrier is like a shield that exists to prevent chemicals and cells in the bloodstream from entering the CNS, while allowing the good stuff to pass through. Magnetic resonance imaging (MRI) shows that when a person with MS is having a relapse, the blood-brain barrier has broken down in the brain or spinal cord. This allows immune cells to cross over and attack the myelin.

Alert

Most people experience their first symptoms of MS between the ages of twenty and forty. Although scientists have documented cases of MS in young children and elderly adults, symptoms rarely begin before age fifteen or after age sixty. The average age of diagnosis is between twenty-nine and thirty-three years of age.

A key player in MS is a white blood cell in the immune system called a T cell. Scientists have learned that when specific T cells become activated, they leave the bloodstream and cross the blood-brain barrier to damage myelin.

Putting It All Together

Although MS is referred to as a neurological disorder, the problem seems to originate with the immune system. Research has shown that some sort of malfunction in the immune system interferes with the functioning of the nervous system. The process seems to follow these steps:

1. A faulty immune system loses the ability to distinguish the good cells from the bad cells.
2. A breakdown in the blood-brain barrier allows immune cells to travel into the CNS to attack the myelin and axons.
3. Toxic substances are released into the CNS, causing inflammation and resulting in the breakdown of myelin (in a process called demyelination) and axons.
4. Scar tissue forms where nervous system damage has occurred.
5. The inflammation, demyelination, and broken axons cause the nerve impulses to be slowed down in the transmission process, resulting in neurological symptoms.
6. The body tries to heal some of the damage caused by this process by naturally reducing inflammation and doing its best to regenerate myelin.

A useful way to picture the process of MS is to imagine a lamp cord. The electrical wire within the lamp cord is protected by a plastic coating, just as myelin coats and protects the nerves. Now, imagine that some kind of incident occurs that damages the cord in several small places. When you turn on the lamp, the electrical current may be disrupted, resulting in a faulty lamp. This is similar to what happens during an attack (or an exacerbation). Perhaps you grab a roll of electrical tape and try to patch up areas of damage on the cord, which is similar to what happens in remyelination. Now imagine further that the cord is somehow severed. In MS, broken or severed axons are no longer able to transmit a signal.

Essential

Repairing damaged myelin is the focus of the Myelin Repair Foundation, an organization whose aim is to accelerate research for myelin repair. Repairing the myelin damaged by MS may improve signal transmission in the central nervous system and reduce the symptoms of the disease. For more information visit *www.myelinrepair.org*.

Suspected Causes of MS

Although thousands of researchers across the world are trying to solve the puzzle, the exact cause of MS remains a mystery. Current research suggests that several factors may play a role in its development, including genetics and something in a person's environment, possibly a virus.

Genetic Factors

Genetic factors probably play a role in making someone susceptible to MS, but it is currently believed that no single gene is responsible for causing it. This is known as genetic predisposition and is different from a genetic or hereditary illness that is passed directly from parent to child. Evidence suggests that MS occurs often enough in the same families that it is unlikely to be a coincidence. Take a look at the some of the statistics:

- The risk of developing MS is higher if another family member is affected, so if your brother, sister, parent, or child has MS, you have a 1 to 3 percent chance of developing it yourself.

- An identical twin runs a 30 percent chance of acquiring MS if her twin has the disease, whereas a nonidentical twin has only a 4 percent chance if her twin has it.
- In the United States the prevalence of MS is higher in Caucasians than in other racial groups. Caucasians have twice the incidence rates of African Americans.
- The higher prevalence of MS among people of northern European background suggests some genetic susceptibility. Native Indians of North and South America, the Japanese, and other Asian peoples have very low incidence rates.

These statistics suggest that genetic factors play a role in MS, but other data point to triggers in the environment. Some researchers feel that MS develops because a person is genetically more likely to react to something in the environment. Then when she comes in contact with that agent, it triggers the immune system to attack the CNS. Sophisticated new techniques for identifying genes may help answer questions about the role of genetics in the development of MS.

Environmental Factors

Environmental factors associated with MS only serve to deepen the mystery, as several interesting patterns have been discovered by researchers over the years.

MS is several times more prevalent in temperate climates, so those living farthest away from the equator have a higher risk of developing the disease. A map of the United States shows that the prevalence of MS increases in northern latitudes, where the occurrence of MS is significantly higher than that observed in southern states such as Florida. This might indicate some triggering factor in the environment, such as toxins or vitamin deficiencies, causing MS to manifest in those whose immune systems are genetically predisposed to it.

Studies are now under way to determine if a lack of vitamin D may play a role, as natural sunlight is responsible for the manufacturing of the vitamin in your body. The findings may help explain why both MS and rheumatoid arthritis are more common in northern climates, where sunlight is often scarce.

Migration patterns also seem to play a role in the development of MS. Studies have shown that those who live in areas of the world with a high risk of MS and then move to an area with a low incidence before they turn fifteen years old have a lower risk of developing the disease. This data may suggest that exposure to some unknown environmental agent before puberty may predispose someone to develop MS at a later time.

Scientists periodically receive reports of "MS clusters." The most infamous case took place in the Faeroe Islands north of Scotland in the years following the arrival of British troops during World War II. Despite years of study of this and other clusters, scientists have not been able to pinpoint a direct environmental factor.

Fact

Researchers believe that the cause of MS cannot be entirely environmental, because different racial groups living together do not have the same rates of incidence. Scotland reports one of the highest incidence rates of MS: one in every 500. The incidence rate in the United States is roughly one in every 700.

Gender Differences

By most recent studies, it appears that women are two to three times more likely to develop MS than men. The ratio of women to men may be increasing, since studies several decades ago indicated that the ratio of women to men was about two to one.

Scientists are looking for possible reasons for the increase, including lifestyle choices and environmental triggers, but one interesting target of research is hormones. Young women tend to acquire autoimmune diseases at a higher rate than young men—perhaps because men's testosterone levels are high enough to prevent these diseases.

Studies have also shown that women have fewer relapses during pregnancy, suggesting estrogen, progesterone, or other pregnancy-related hormones may play a stabilizing role in pregnant women.

Essential

Researchers are currently looking at estriol—a female sex hormone—to see what role it plays in decreasing the activity of MS during pregnancy. A study by UCLA neuroscientists showed that estriol in oral tablet form can decrease the size and number of brain lesions, and increase protective immune responses in patients with relapsing-remitting MS.

Viral Causes

One of the top suspects for triggering MS is a viral agent, and yet, after years of research, one specific virus has not emerged as a proven trigger. Viruses seem like a good candidate because the immune response to viruses may cause demyelinating disease in humans and animals. Proteins of some viruses are similar to those of myelin, and some scientists theorize that this may cause confusion in the immune system, causing the immune cells to attack their own protein as well as that of the virus.

Scientists speculate that an infectious agent almost everyone has come in contact with may cause an abnormal reaction in the immune system in people who are already at risk of developing the disease. Some studies have suggested that many viruses such as measles, herpes, and the flu viruses may be associated with MS. To date, however, this belief has not been proven.

Here are the primary suspects:

Human Herpesvirus 6 (HHV-6)

Herpes virus 6 is a common virus that causes a condition in young children known as roseola. Some studies indicate that HHV-6 infection may play a role in MS.

Epstein-Barr Virus (EBV)

Evidence suggests an association between EBV, the cause of mononucleosis, and MS. Like HHV-6, EBV is an extremely common virus. Nearly all people have been exposed to EBV. Some researchers propose that people with MS have an atypical immune response to EBV, and this response may increase the risk of MS.

Chlamydia Pneumoniae

This atypical bacteria has been associated with persistent inflammation. A few studies have reported significantly higher rates of previous chlamydia infection in patients with MS than in individuals without MS. Other viruses that have been investigated include measles virus, adenovirus, and the retroviruses (HIV, HTLV-I, and HTLV-II), but none have emerged as having any definitive importance at this time.

New Treatments and Choices

Despite the challenges in targeting the cause of MS, the good news is that science continues to unravel the mysteries of the disease and more is known today about MS than ever before. People with MS now have a near-normal life expectancy.

The years between 1990 and 1999 were termed "The Decade of the Brain," an initiative designated by Congress to enhance public awareness of the brain through research and study. MS benefited enormously through these efforts, giving rise to a new sense of hope and optimism. Advances were made on many fronts, including diagnosis, symptom management, and new drug therapies.

Magnetic Resonance Imaging

Sophisticated new techniques applied to MRI have allowed earlier detection of MS scarring or plaques, resulting in a quicker diagnosis. MRI studies also confirmed that the disease remains active even when patients feel no symptoms, underscoring the need for earlier treatment and close monitoring of the disease.

Gene Research

In 2007, a large-scale genomic study uncovered new genetic variations associated with MS, findings that suggest a possible link between MS and other autoimmune diseases. The study, led by an international consortium of clinical scientists and genomics experts, was the first comprehensive study investigating the genetic basis of MS.

Two genetic regions were identified—the IL-2 receptor and the IL-7 receptor—and both are expected to become major focal points of research. Current genomic studies are helping to pinpoint genes that may elevate the risk of developing MS, pointing the way to new areas of research and new therapeutic targets to both treat and eventually prevent MS.

Information Highway

Computer technology has allowed MS researchers from all over the world to collect and share information, helping to isolate and identify characteristic patterns of MS. Computers have also served to empower people with MS. Research and support are just one click away, giving people access to treatment information, research studies, and the opportunity to find support in the global community.

New Drugs and Therapies

New drugs and therapies have been introduced to help treat the underlying disease process as well as symptoms of the disease. Those that treat the disease process are known as disease-modifying therapies (DMTs) while those that alleviate symptoms are known as symptomatic therapies. There are currently six FDA-approved disease-modifying medications for MS.

Fact

According to the National MS Society (NMSS), there are more potential drugs in the pipeline for MS than ever before. Each year, thousands of research articles are published, probing the causes of MS and potential treatment strategies. There are also exciting new areas of research in cell biology, genetics, and stem cells.

Although no one can predict when, or if, there will be a cure for MS, there is good reason to be hopeful about the future. The ongoing advances in research are occurring at a faster rate than ever before and continue to add to our understanding of how MS works and progresses. Researchers are already looking ahead to the next generation of treatments and, hopefully, a cure.

CHAPTER 2

Signs and Symptoms

IF ONE THING is for certain in this rather puzzling disease, it's that MS is as varied and unique as the person who has it. Just as there are no two people who are exactly alike in the world, neither will any two people experience MS in quite the same way. This is because no two people have myelin or axon damage in exactly the same places in their CNS and because individual immune systems vary. The symptoms of MS, therefore, differ greatly from person to person, and your particular symptoms are unique to you.

Disease Types in MS

In order to understand the way the symptoms behave in MS, it is important to understand the four disease types, which is a way of categorizing the various patterns of the disease.

Relapsing-Remitting MS (RRMS)

The vast majority of people (85 percent) presenting with MS are first diagnosed with RRMS. RRMS is characterized by periods of worsening (caused by acute inflammation) in which, typically, new symptoms appear. The relapses are followed by periods of remission, during which time the person fully or partially recovers.

Secondary Progressive MS (SPMS)

In this form of MS, a person who initially had relapsing-remitting MS begins to develop a slowly progressive worsening of neurological function, especially leg strength and walking ability. Within ten years, about 50 percent of people with RRMS will transition to SPMS.

Primary Progressive MS (PPMS)

This type of MS is characterized by a gradual progression of the disease from its onset with no remissions at all. About 10 percent of MS patients are in this category.

Progressive-Relapsing MS (PRMS)

This form of MS follows a progressive course from onset, punctuated by relapses. There is significant recovery immediately following a relapse, but between relapses there is a gradual worsening of symptoms. This form of MS is rare, accounting for only 5 percent of MS patients.

Fact

Other categories include malignant MS and benign MS. Malignant MS, which is also sometimes known as Marburg's variant, is characterized by an extremely aggressive course of the disease. It is extremely rare. Benign MS is considered a subgroup of RRMS and is characterized by a person who has had MS for fifteen or more years with few relapses and little, if any, disability.

You may note that RRMS and SPMS are not different diseases or different types of disease, but are, in fact, time points of the same disease. RRMS transitions into SPMS for a percentage of people with MS.

Since MS is so unpredictable, it is impossible to predict how the disease course will go in any one person. Thus, it is recommended that anyone diagnosed with the disease begin drug therapy right away.

The Symptoms of MS

Symptoms are the complaints that you bring to your doctor's office and signs are the clues your doctor discovers through examination. Together, symptoms and signs are termed findings. It is the role of the physician to find physical signs that substantiate a patient's complaints or symptoms, but symptoms can exist in the absence of signs. You may have tingling or numbness in your hand that your doctor can't substantiate on examination. Other times, your doctor may find signs upon neurological examination for which you are not experiencing symptoms. You may have optic neuritis (inflammation of the optic nerve), and not note any visual difficulties.

Alert

There are a number of diseases that only cause mild or vague symptoms, especially at first. People may not even feel abnormal, but have a vague feeling that things are not quite right. They may feel unusually tired, for example, or have intermittent numbness in a limb. In some conditions, the symptoms get worse over time, but in others, the symptoms may stay vague for a time. This often happens in the early stages of MS. Any symptom needs checking with your doctor, even if it seems mild or minor.

The symptoms of MS include fatigue, weakness, numbness, cognitive difficulties, clumsiness of fine motor coordination, and bowel or bladder problems, to name a few.

MS symptoms generally appear between the ages of twenty and forty. The onset of MS may be dramatic or so mild that a person doesn't even notice any symptoms until later in the course of the disease.

As you learned in Chapter 1, disruption of communication between the brain and other parts of the body prevent normal passage of sensations and messages, leading to the symptoms of MS. The demyelinated areas appear as plaques (or scars). The progression of symptoms in MS is caused by the development of new plaques in the portion of the brain or spinal cord that controls the affected areas. Since there is no evidence that there is any pattern to the development of new plaques, the progression of MS is unpredictable.

In Chapter 9, the symptoms of MS will be fleshed out further. In this chapter, the symptoms most people experience in the beginning stages of the disease will be discussed.

It's very important to remember that you will not experience all of the symptoms that are addressed here.

While most any symptom can appear to signal a problem that may prompt you to call your physician, the most common problems people bring to their doctor's office for the first time include the following:

- Tingling
- Numbness
- Loss of balance
- Weakness in one or more limbs
- Blurred or double vision

Less common first symptoms of MS include slurred speech, weakness, lack of coordination, and cognitive difficulties. As the disease progresses, other symptoms may include muscle spasms, sensitivity to heat, fatigue, changes in thinking or perception, and sexual disturbances.

Most people with MS will experience more than one symptom, and though there are symptoms common to many people, no person will have all of them. The good news is that your doctor can help you keep your symptoms under control.

Some symptoms come and go while others may be permanent. Most people with MS are on very intimate terms with their symptoms and use them as a yardstick to assess their current level of health as it pertains to the disease. For example, if you have overtaxed yourself, an old friend—such as numbness in your hand—may show up to remind you to take it easy for a while. This is sometimes referred to as "fluctuation of a chronic symptom" and is usually *not* due to new disease activity. In contrast, entirely new symptoms, especially those that are notable enough to interfere with day-to-day functioning, usually indicate that you are experiencing an exacerbation. As a result, you should always report new symptoms to your doctor.

Question

Do MS symptoms follow a typical pattern?
Symptoms of MS may be mild or severe, of long duration or short, and they may appear in various combinations, depending on the area of the nervous system affected. Complete or partial remission of symptoms, especially in the early stages of the disease, occurs in approximately 70 percent of MS patients.

Visual Disturbances

Problems with vision are relatively common in MS. MS may cause blurring of vision or difficulty with eye movement.

Optic Neuritis

Optic neuritis is the most common problem in MS. Almost 70 percent of people with MS experience optic neuritis at some point during the course of the disease and, in fact, 35 percent visit their doctor with optic neuritis presenting as an initial symptom.

The rate of onset of optic neuritis can vary from a few hours to a few days and sometimes greater. Often, sight is at its worst about one week after onset of symptoms. The good news is that optic neuritis is transient and often occurs in just one eye, and any vision loss is usually temporary.

Diplopia

Diplopia refers to double vision. In MS, the nerve pathways that control eye movements may be damaged. When this occurs, the eyes may not move through their full range of movement and double vision may occur.

Nystagmus

Nystagmus is defined as jerky, involuntary movement of the eyes and is usually related to brain stem inflammation in areas that control eye movement. Nystagmus may be vertical or horizontal and can occur in one or both eyes. Loss of balance or dizziness may accompany this symptom.

Afferent Pupillary Defect (APD)

Afferent pupillary defect occurs when one pupil fails to dilate properly. It doesn't cause visual disturbances, so you may not notice this yourself unless someone points it out to you. In people with MS, it usually happens because the person has had optic neuritis, even if the episode was so mild that he was not aware that it occurred. APD is identified by examining the eyes with a bright light. During a neurological exam, your doctor may perform the swinging flashlight test, where your doctor shines a flashlight in one eye and then the other. In normal circumstances, when a light is shined in one eye, both pupils constrict (get smaller) at the same time. However, when a light is shined in the affected eye of a patient with APD, the pupil of the affected eye dilates (gets larger) rather than constricts.

Sensory Symptoms

While sensory symptoms can be aggravating, they are not life-threatening and can usually be managed or treated. These symptoms are very common in MS and include feelings of burning, aching, and tingling discomfort most often in the limbs.

Paresthesias

Paresthesias, which are characterized by tingling, numbness, itching, burning, or stabbing or tearing pain, occur in up to 55 percent of people with MS and may be the earliest MS symptom.

Lhermitte's Sign

Lhermitte's sign describes the electric buzzing sensations in the limbs and torso brought on by movement of the neck and is most often triggered by lowering the chin to touch the chest. Lhermitte's is an indicator of lesions in the cervical spine. Movement of the neck causes the damaged nerves to be stretched and send erroneous signals to the brain.

Trigeminal Neuralgia (TN)

Trigeminal neuralgia is an acute, shocklike pain in the regions of the face served by the trigeminal nerve. This nerve serves three areas of the face: the forehead, cheek, and jaw. TN can affect some or all of these areas (usually on one side of the face) and can be triggered by a number of factors, including crying, laughing, or brushing one's teeth.

Motor Symptoms

Motor symptoms in MS are extremely variable and can range from slight weakness and a lack of coordination to loss of control over one or more muscle groups.

Babinski Reflex

The Babinski reflex is a neurological sign in MS in which stroking the outside sole of the foot with a pointed object causes an upward (extensor) movement of the big toe rather than the normal (flexor) bunching and downward movement of the toes. This reflex is normal in younger children, but abnormal after the age of two.

Spasticity

Spasticity is a condition in which muscle tone becomes greatly increased. Muscle tone is what enables people to move limbs or hold a position. The term refers to the level of tension or resistance to movement in a muscle. For instance, to bend your arm, you must shorten or contract the biceps muscle at the front of the arm (increasing the tone) and at the same time lengthen or relax the triceps muscle at the back of the arm (reducing the tone). When someone has spasticity in a limb, the signals from the brain are altered in such a way that opposing muscles, such as the biceps and triceps, may be simultaneously shortened or contracted. This causes the affected limb to feel stiff or tight and to be resistant to movement. Aching muscles and muscle spasms and cramps are also a common problem in MS.

Dysarthria

Dysarthria refers to speech problems. In MS, dysarthria may be caused by decreased function of the nerves that control the muscles involved with speaking. Dysarthria may be characterized by slurred speech, lack or articulation, or altered rate of speech.

Paresis

Paresis is the term used to describe muscle weakness, a common symptom of MS that is caused by lesions along the pathway of the nerves that control muscle movement. Muscle weakness can cause problems with walking and coordination.

Ataxia

Ataxia is the inability to coordinate voluntary muscle movements. A person with ataxia will appear to be unsteady when walking or off-balance when standing. There are three types of ataxia: Cerebellar ataxia is caused by lesions in the cerebellum and causes incoordination of extremity or eye movements or incoordination of speech. Vestibular ataxia is caused by lesions to the brain stem and can result in loss of balance or dizziness. Sensory ataxia is caused by damage to position-sensing nerves and causes the brain to be confused as to the positioning of the limbs.

Fatigue

Fatigue is one of the most common symptoms in MS and the majority of people with MS experience it at one time or another. MS fatigue is different than normal fatigue and science has not yet been able to explain what causes it.

Some of the fatigue people with MS experience might be caused by sleep disruption from a malfunctioning bladder, or perhaps from expending a lot of energy completing tasks—such as getting dressed—when they are experiencing muscle weakness. Other possible causes of fatigue are depression, medications, or other medical conditions, such as anemia and thyroid disease. But beyond these causes, there does seem to be an MS-related fatigue that often gets worse as the day progresses, is more severe than normal fatigue, and occurs whether or not you've had a good night's sleep.

Eighty to ninety percent of people with MS report fatigue as a symptom. For about two-thirds, fatigue sometimes limits daily activities.

Essential

Cognitive fatigue (also known as mental fatigue) is also common in MS, making it difficult for some people to sustain concentration over a long period of time. One recent study evaluated cognitive fatigue in MS. Declines in memory and planning ability were seen in people with MS who were given a math test, while volunteers without MS had improvement in these areas when the test was administered again.

Cognitive Symptoms

Cognition is another word for thinking. It was once believed that cognitive symptoms in MS were uncommon, but in the last ten years or so, researchers have learned that cognition can indeed be affected by the disease. People with MS often report having trouble coming up with a word in conversation or remembering things, such as items to purchase at the grocery store. About one-half of people with MS have cognitive difficulties. However, for the majority of these people, thinking problems are mild. It is believed that those who have a large number of lesions in their brain are more at risk for experiencing cognitive difficulties. Here are some of the cognitive symptoms seen in MS:

- Problems with memory
- Problems with concentration
- Problems with planning and problem solving
- Problems with visuospatial skills
- Slower processing of thoughts

Cognitive deficits are more common in people who have changes in the cerebrum than in people who have changes in the cerebellum, brain stem, and spinal cord alone.

Bladder and Bowel Problems

While bladder and bowel problems are fairly common in MS, doctors have quite a few tricks up their sleeves to help control them, including medications and self-help strategies. Symptoms such as urinary frequency or retention can occur, along with urinary tract infections. About 85 percent of people with MS are likely to experience these problems, which can occur early in the disease or late, although bowel and bladder dysfunction is rarely the first symptom in MS. Keep in mind that like other MS symptoms, bladder problems can vary from person to person. The most common bladder problem is called "spastic bladder." This is when the bladder is unable to hold the normal amount of urine or does not empty properly.

Bowel problems include constipation or urgency. Constipation is very common among people with MS and can be blamed on a lack of physical activity or the medications you may be taking to manage your MS. Depression can also affect the digestive system. Urgency is characterized by a feeling of "having to go right now!" Causes can vary from long-term constipation to nerve damage or overuse of laxatives.

Bowel problems can also stem from a neurologic disturbance caused by an interruption of impulses to the brain that signal the need for a bowel movement. This book will take another look at bowel and bladder symptoms in Chapter 9, but for now it's good to note that these sorts of problems are often easily managed and controlled.

Less Common Symptoms

There are other symptoms—though rare—that you should be aware of. You're not likely to come across them on many lists, but knowing that they are included in the symptom spectrum is important. Less recognized symptoms include:

- Headache
- Hearing problems
- Vertigo
- Sleep disorders
- Seizures

Both doctors and patients should be aware that these symptoms can be related to MS, and can typically be controlled with the proper treatment.

All of the symptoms of MS can be distressing, but some cause more trouble than others. It's important to remember, though, that many people with MS do not experience severe enough symptoms to significantly restrict their daily lives.

Alert

Some symptoms of MS may be worsened by increased body temperature, which may be provoked by fever, intense physical activity, or exposure to sun, hot baths, or showers. This worsening of symptoms does not qualify as a true relapse. Once the body's temperature returns to normal, the heat-provoked symptoms typically disappear.

Visible and Invisible MS

MS symptoms can be thought of as visible or invisible. Visible symptoms are the symptoms that other people can see; in this case, it is obvious to others that the person with MS is having difficulty. Visible symptoms include problems with walking, eye function, weakness, or coordination. Invisible symptoms are symptoms that only the patient is aware of. They are not obvious to others—sometimes not even to the health care professional. Invisible symptoms include cognitive problems, pain, depression, fatigue, mood changes, and sensory symptoms such as numbness or tingling. Bowel and bladder problems can also be invisible symptoms.

Essential

Invisible symptoms can complicate the lives of people with MS. Despite how he appears on the outside, the person may be experiencing significant difficulty on the inside. He may be having a hard time getting family members or coworkers to understand how he feels. It's important to teach others how to respect your limitations and acknowledge what you are experiencing. It's also important to share your invisible symptoms with your health care team.

Although there are more than fifty symptoms included in the MS spectrum, most people will experience relatively few of those on the list. Symptoms are effectively controlled by medications, rehabilitation, and other management strategies. Being proactive about symptoms can help avoid unnecessary complications and improve the quality of your life. You'll look more closely at symptom management in Chapter 9.

CHAPTER 3

The Diagnosis Process

WHILE DIAGNOSING MS has come a long way in recent years, it is not an exact science. That's because there is no definitive test to determine if someone has MS. A diagnosis is based on a number of factors, including patient history, a neurological exam, and the results of diagnostic tests such as magnetic resonance imaging (MRI). If you arrive at your primary care doctor's office with certain neurological symptoms in tow—say, fatigue as well as numbness in your left hand—you may be referred to a neurologist, a doctor who diagnoses and treats neurological disorders.

Differential Diagnosis

If your neurologist suspects MS, she'll probably schedule a battery of tests that may help confirm her suspicions. While this may sound pretty straightforward, getting a firm diagnosis can be a frustrating process for some. One reason is that MS can mimic other diseases and they must first be excluded. This is called a *differential diagnosis*—a list of diseases that are similar to MS that must be ruled out by your doctor.

Since there are many potential symptoms associated with MS, there are a large number of conditions that are clinically similar. A few of the diseases that have similar symptoms to MS include:

- **Lyme disease.** An infection caused by bacteria that is carried by deer ticks. Lyme disease can cause symptoms similar to MS, including fatigue, muscle weakness, and sensory symptoms such as pins and needles sensations.
- **Vitamin B12 deficiency.** A deficiency of vitamin B12 in the body can cause multiple neurological symptoms including numbness and tingling in the hands and feet, fatigue, and muscle weakness.
- **Acute disseminated encephalomyelitis (ADEM).** A demyelinating neurological disease characterized by inflammation of the brain and spinal cord. ADEM is characterized as an autoimmune disease.
- **Sarcoidosis.** A disease that causes inflammation in the tissues of multiple organs, including the brain and spinal cord.
- **Sjögren's syndrome.** An autoimmune disease in which the immune system of the body attacks its own moisture producing glands. CNS symptoms may include fatigue, weakness, and walking difficulty.
- **Lupus.** An autoimmune disease that can cause inflammation and damage to almost any part of the body, including the heart, lungs, kidneys, blood vessels, or brain. As with MS, symptoms may come and go.

In addition to this list, there are other diseases that mimic MS; in fact, as many as 10 percent of people diagnosed with the disease actually have another condition, including strokes, tumors, and the diseases and disorders mentioned above. Once your neurologist has ruled them out—performed the necessary tests to exclude them from the list—she may conduct procedures that often help in pinpointing MS. These include obtaining a thorough medical history from the patient, imaging techniques, lumbar punctures, evoked potentials (a test that measures the time it takes for nerves to respond to stimulation), and laboratory examination of blood samples.

Your Medical History

Obtaining a thorough medical history is part of the diagnostic process. A talented neurologist can extract clues during a question-and-answer period with you that may help determine if your symptoms are following a specific pattern. Many people who are diagnosed with MS can remember a time—perhaps a few months or years before—when similar symptoms arose that they ignored. "Well, yes," they might say, "a few years ago I had numbness in my foot, but it went away after a few days and I didn't think much of it." Sharing anything significant in your medical history will be very helpful to your doctor. Information from a patient's history can help localize a lesion, and a diagnostic test (such as an MRI) can be directed to evaluate the suspicious area. A complete medical history includes the following:

- Your current symptoms
- Symptoms similar to those you are experiencing that may have occurred in the past
- Past illnesses and the treatment you received
- Past surgeries
- Any accidents you might have had
- Medication use
- Any allergies you have
- Your use of tobacco, alcohol, and recreational drugs
- The medical histories of your family and their causes of death

It's a good idea to come to your appointment with a written list of symptoms, family health history, and other pertinent information. Thinking things through beforehand will ensure that anything important is included in your discussion with your physician.

Essential

> Keeping a medical journal is a good idea. You can record and keep track of your symptoms, detail visits to your health care provider, and record test results. Journaling is a great way to track your medical information as well as vent your personal feelings. Keeping up with the details of your life (both medical and nonmedical) can give you a sense of control.

Neurological Exam

Before the advent of the MRI, the neurological exam allowed astute physicians to pinpoint a lesion in the CNS, often with great accuracy. It is very rare to be diagnosed with MS based solely on a neurological exam these days; other tests, such as MRIs, lumbar puncture, or evoked potentials, are used to complete the picture.

In its most basic form, the neurological exam is a test that measures how well your nervous system is working, specifically the areas where nervous system function has decreased. The test is not only given in the diagnostic stage but also repeated throughout the course of the disease. People who have had MS for a period of time are very familiar with neurological exams.

During the exam, the neurologist will test your reflexes, vision, strength, and coordination; note the speed and agility as you walk; look for changes in sensitivity to touch; and check for any problems with talking or swallowing. Some of the signs the neurologist is looking for are things you may not have noticed yourself; perhaps upon examination one of your eyes has signs of optic neuritis although you hadn't noticed anything wrong. Another sign that may be picked up during a neurological exam is the presence of the Babinski reflex (see Chapter 2). Again, this is something that you might not notice yourself, but may be an indication that all is not well with your CNS.

Fact

The neurological examination is divided into several components, each focusing on a different part of the nervous system: mental status, cranial nerves, motor system, sensory system, deep tendon reflexes, coordination of the cerebellum, and gait. The exam requires skill, patience, and intelligence on the part of the physician to determine if there is a problem in your central nervous system.

Imaging Techniques

The development of magnetic resonance imaging in the late 1970s provided a breakthrough of sorts for MS professionals and patients alike. Peering into the brain and spinal cord became possible without risk of injury to the patient. It has also allowed researchers to better understand the role of plaques or lesions in the disease process and to monitor disease activity. MRI has also been helpful in measuring the effectiveness of drug therapies for MS.

MRIs have become an important tool in diagnosing the disease, allowing doctors to identify telltale lesions in the brains and spinal cords of patients who are suspected of having MS. But the complexities of MS prevent the MRI from being a perfect diagnostic indicator. Lesions can appear in the brains of people who do not have MS, and research indicates that about 5 percent of people with MS may have a normal MRI—especially in the early stages of the disease.

MRIs are safe for almost everyone, but it is important to tell your doctor or technician if you have any implant devices, including cochlear implants, a pacemaker, pumps (such as an insulin pump) or metal stabilization rods, plates, or screws from surgery. Not all implant devices are a problem, so don't assume that an MRI is ruled out if you have one.

You will also want to convey whether you are, or may be, pregnant, have tattoos (some tattoos contain metal), wear an intrauterine device, wear dentures, or have been exposed to metal fragments from a war wound or from work in construction.

Question

How do MRIs target MS?
MRI uses extremely powerful magnetic fields to examine specific compounds, such as water, in the body's tissues. MS lesions have higher than normal water content that can be identified by the MRI, which pinpoints the areas of damage. MRI scans are much more detailed than CT (computerized tomography) scans and x-rays, especially of tissues that are not bone, such as the brain and spinal cord.

As noted, a contrast material called gadolinium—a dye— is delivered by intravenous infusion during the scan. The contrast is used to highlight new or active areas of inflammation in the CNS caused by a breakdown of the blood-brain barrier. How does it work? The gadolinium tends to accumulate in new plaques. The plaques are enhanced by the contrast (or dye) used in MRI. It helps your health care provider separate active lesions from the normal parts of the brain. (Old plaques do not typically enhance with gadolinium.)

Essential

It is important to make an appointment with your neurologist to discuss the results of your MRI. The doctor will be able to tell you what sort of changes—if any—have occurred in your brain or spinal cord. The time you take to review your MRIs and ask questions helps you to establish a relationship with your doctor and allows you to take an active role in your care.

Your doctor may order more than one MRI at first—one with contrast and one without. If you are pregnant, or suspect that you are pregnant, it is important to discuss this with your doctor ahead of time. When preparing for an MRI, wear comfortable, loose-fitting clothing. You may also be asked to change into a guest robe; clothes often have metallic fibers or fasteners that can interfere with imaging. You'll also be asked to remove jewelry, eyeglasses, and dental implants. It's best to leave valuables at home.

Alert

Patients with kidney problems should talk to their doctors about the use of certain gadolinium-based agents that are used to enhance of the quality of MRI. These patients might be at risk for developing nephrogenic systemic fibrosis, a potentially fatal disease. There is no risk for this condition for people who have normal kidney function.

An MRI looks like a cylindrical tube with a tunnel through the middle. A sliding table moves you into the center of the tube, where you will be asked to hold still while the scans are taken. A loud clicking or banging sound can be heard (about 90 decibels), but earplugs or headphones are given to make the noise less intrusive. You'll be able to communicate with a technician any time the need arises.

(Many people report that they fall asleep during an MRI!) The experience isn't too uncomfortable unless keeping still isn't easy for you. The average time for an MRI scan is about thirty minutes, but the time can vary depending on how many views your doctor has ordered. A radiologist will interpret the results and send a report to your doctor.

Evoked Potentials

An evoked potential measures how long it takes for nerves to respond to stimulation. The response speed in people with MS may be slower, indicating a lesion somewhere in the CNS. The tests measure the electrical activity of the brain in response to stimulation of specific sensory nerve pathways and can help determine a diagnosis of MS. There are three types of evoked potential responses:

- Visual evoked potential (VEP) is measured when the eyes are stimulated with test patterns. A checkerboard pattern on a computer screen or a strobe light might be used.
- Somatosensory evoked potential (SSEP) is measured when the arms or legs are stimulated by a very mild electrical impulse.
- Brain stem auditory evoked potential (BAEP) is measured when the hearing is stimulated by listening to a test tone.

The doctor is looking for both the size of the response and the speed with which the brain receives the signal. Weaker or slow signals may indicate that demyelination has occurred and that MS is a possibility. Each type of response is recorded from brain waves by using electrodes that are taped on the scalp. The placement of the electrodes depends on which potential is being tested. To test visual potential, for example, the electrodes are taped near the back of the head over areas in the brain that are responsible for visual stimuli. Currently, neurologists use the results of the VEP to aid in diagnosing MS as it identifies difficulty in transmission of the vision pathway—a common finding in MS. The results are not specific for MS, so evoked potentials by themselves cannot confirm a diagnosis. Other tests must be performed to complete the clinical picture.

Lumbar Puncture

A lumbar puncture (also called a spinal tap) is a procedure that removes spinal fluid from the spinal canal. Testing the fluid may help your doctor pinpoint MS. Spinal fluid (also called cerebrospinal fluid) is a clear liquid produced in the ventricles of the brain. Its job is to protect and fill the cavities of the brain and spinal cord. The fluid contains sugar, proteins, and other substances that are found in the blood. Tests performed on the spinal fluid look for evidence of inflammation in the CNS. Ninety percent of people with MS have elevated levels of antibodies or specific types of antibodies (called *oligoclonal bands*). Other CNS infections and inflammatory diseases can also cause these tests to be abnormal, so again, the test cannot be used as a definitive indicator of MS.

Question

How do I prepare for a spinal tap?
No special preparations are needed before a spinal tap, which can be performed in your neurologist's office. But you should ask your doctor for specific guidelines about discontinuing alcohol use, aspirin products, or anticoagulant medications before the procedure. Tell your doctor if you have any allergies. It is also helpful to have your doctor explain what he is doing as he performs the procedure as it may serve to reduce your anxiety.

Of all the MS tests, the spinal tap is the most invasive and seems to generate the most anxiety. Although infrequent, complications can occur as a result of the spinal tap. For example, 5 to 30 percent of people who undergo a spinal tap get a headache, commonly referred to as a post-lumbar-puncture headache. Drinking plenty of fluids, especially caffeinated drinks, can help reduce your chances of getting a headache, as will lying flat for up to an hour after the procedure is done.

The procedure takes approximately forty minutes. You will be asked to lie on your side in a fetal position, with your knees drawn as close as possible to your chest. Your neurologist will inject a local anesthetic into your lower back and once you are numb, he will insert a hollow needle into your lower back between two lumbar vertebrae. This may cause some minor discomfort or a slight burning sensation. After the fluid is collected, the needle is removed and a bandage is placed over the area. The site may be a little sore for a day or two.

Diagnostic Criteria

Because there is no one single test that can diagnose MS, doctors rely on evidence gathered from clinical examination, patient history, and the results from various tests. But as the last two decades have brought new technology and a new understanding of the disease, the criteria that doctors use to make a diagnosis have also changed.

In April 2001, an international panel in association with the NMSS recommended revised diagnostic criteria for MS. These new criteria have become known as the McDonald criteria after their lead author, Dr. W. I. McDonald. They make use of advances in MRI imaging techniques and were intended to replace the twenty-year-old Poser criteria.

It is helpful to understand the criteria that doctors use to make an MS diagnosis as it explains what your doctor is looking for and why—in some cases—a definite diagnosis is delayed. In the past, the basic criteria for an MS diagnosis were:

- There must be objective evidence of two relapses, where new symptoms appear or prior symptoms become worse for at least twenty-four hours.

- The two relapses must be separated in time by at least one month. And they must show evidence of having occurred in different areas of the CNS.
- There must be no other explanation for the symptoms.

With the recently developed McDonald criteria, doctors can utilize new diagnostic tools, especially MRIs, to make an MS diagnosis. The need for a speedy and accurate diagnosis is especially important, since disease-modifying drugs are available.

The Importance of Early Diagnosis and Treatment

Several important developments in the field of MS research have served to underscore the need for early diagnosis, specifically the disease-modifying therapies (DMTs) along with a more thorough understanding of what happens between relapses.

Through the use of MRI, researchers now understand that the disease may actually be active during periods of apparent remission. In other words, during a remission, when your symptoms are silent or have improved—when you think the disease is stable—the disease process may still be active in your CNS.

Alert

Studies support the idea that early treatment is imperative. According to the American Academy of Neurology, early treatment can significantly delay the initial progression of MS. And since the DMTs target inflammation, treatment in the early stages (when inflammation is at its worst) is more effective.

Researchers are studying what are called clinically silent lesions—lesions that don't cause obvious symptoms but are nonetheless actively damaging your CNS. In fact, researchers agree that many patients have silent lesions years before obvious symptoms begin to surface. As a result, damage to the nervous system can be much more extensive than a health professional might have guessed by just looking at a patient's symptoms or neurological examination. In fact, this unchecked disease activity might surface one day as clinical symptoms and eventually disability. What causes silent lesions? Researchers theorize that some of the lesions that occur in the CNS are located in areas that do not cause obvious symptoms, such as optic neuritis or left-handed weakness.

It wasn't long ago that early diagnosis had little to offer the person with MS, but experts now agree that DMTs (including Avonex, Betaseron, Copaxone, Novantrone, Rebif, and Tysabri) hold the best chance of keeping the disease at bay when started early. Neurologists and researchers alike have been debating the benefits of early treatment in people who have had only one attack and do not fit the criteria for definite MS diagnosis. This is referred to as a clinically isolated syndrome (CIS), which in essence is like a first attack of MS—a single clinical event that points to demyelination in the brain or spinal cord. You may have had, for example, just one single episode of optic neuritis without any other symptoms present. This would constitute a clinically isolated syndrome.

People who have experienced a CIS and have an abnormal MRI are at significant risk for developing MS. Studies that involved the drugs Avonex, Betaseron, and Rebif found that each drug delayed the onset of full MS in people who had experienced their first attack. Treating CIS should be discussed in detail with one's physician. It's a good idea to be well informed so that you can make the decision that is best for you.

The Delayed Diagnosis: Now What?

Even though the MRI has come a long way in helping to diagnose MS more efficiently, it's not uncommon to wait months, even years, for a definite diagnosis. That's because not everyone's symptoms and signs fall within the parameters of the McDonald criteria.

Investigators are continuing their search for a definitive test for MS. Until one is developed, however, evidence of both multiple attacks and CNS lesions must be found before a doctor can make a definite diagnosis.

 Fact

For 10 to 15 percent of those in the diagnosis process, a definite diagnosis is not possible. Over time, with periodic examinations and by monitoring the changes in a person's condition, diagnosis is possible in the vast majority of cases. One recent survey conducted by the NMSS and Teva Neuroscience showed that in a study of almost 2,000 people with MS, it took 37 percent six months or less to receive a definitive diagnosis of MS after their symptoms started.

Your neurologist may take a wait-and-see approach and will continue to follow up with you until it's possible to paint a better clinical picture through office visits and repeat MRIs. For some patients, the wait can be difficult. Uncertain of what is causing their symptoms, they can find the feeling of being in limbo unsettling. Rest assured, your health care professionals are just as eager to pinpoint the cause as you are, but getting an accurate diagnosis is important. You may also want to seek out a second opinion.

Alert

If you have received an uncertain diagnosis, use this time to make some lifestyle changes. Taking good care of your body right now is just as important as it is for someone who has received a definite diagnosis. Strive to live a healthier lifestyle with a nutritious diet and a regular exercise program.

You may also want to spend some time familiarizing yourself with MS by researching drug therapies, checking in with your local chapter of the NMSS, or joining a support group. Keep in mind that most services available for people with MS are also extended to those with possible MS.

When you consider the fact that people were once diagnosed with MS by being placed in a tub of hot water (based on the knowledge that heat exacerbated symptoms), it's easy to appreciate the advancements science has made in diagnosing MS. Without a single "gold standard" diagnostic test, though, MS can still be a difficult disease to pinpoint. The importance of a good physician and adequate testing (not to mention patience) cannot be stressed enough.

Since the new disease-modifying therapies have been introduced, a speedy diagnosis is considered critical, but accuracy is also imperative. New diagnostic tools are currently in the pipeline and may someday make the diagnosis of this complex disease less challenging.

CHAPTER 4

Dealing with a Diagnosis

RECEIVING A DIAGNOSIS of MS is a life-changing event, and feeling overwhelmed by the news is very common. There is certainly no right or wrong way to handle a diagnosis. Some people might prefer to go to bed and curl up under the covers as the news sinks in, while others may be challenged to turn on their computers and look at research studies. Some people even feel a sense of relief at knowing what they're dealing with. People who are newly diagnosed often worry about their future—their jobs, their family, and other important relationships. Learning to deal with a chronic disease is a process, and one that is best dealt with one small step at a time.

Lighten the Load

Feeling overwhelmed by your diagnosis is a natural response. The unknown can conjure up all sorts of doubts and fears about the future. If one thing is for sure, it is that you have more questions than answers right now: What sort of course will my MS take? Will the role I play in my family change? How will I tell my children? How do I make room for this disease in my life?

While these are all important questions, the good news is that they don't all have to be answered today. Taking it one step at a time and breaking up the "big picture" into easy and manageable tasks will help reduce stress and make the coming days easier to handle. You'll need time to cope with the emotional and mental adjustments. Go easy on yourself initially. Cancel an appointment, have dinner delivered, or meet a friend for coffee. You don't have to grapple with the big questions all at once. They'll still be there tomorrow.

Some people may feel relieved when they are diagnosed because they've finally found an explanation for some of the symptoms that have been plaguing them. They've been aware that something is wrong, but their complaints have been dismissed or attributed to something else, such as stress. It is empowering for some people to finally get an answer and take advantage of the treatments and resources available to them. Becoming aware of your condition allows you to take an active part in your treatment and plan for your future.

The Grieving Process

Most everyone is familiar with the five stages of grief outlined by Dr. Elisabeth Kübler-Ross, which has served as a model for under-standing the process by which people deal with tragedy and grief. These stages apply to any form of personal loss, whether it's the loss of a job, the death of a family member, or the diagnosis of an illness. We have all grieved various things in our lives to some extent, especially those things that have created unforeseen changes in our daily routines, such as losing a job or ending a relationship. Grieving the change in the status of your health is perfectly normal—even healthy. Acceptance comes by strapping on your boots and wading through the waters of your fears and uncertainty. Not everyone goes through each stage of grief outlined here or even in the prescribed order. Everyone deals with grief in his or her own way.

Denial

Denial is nature's way of letting in only what you can handle. When someone is in denial, she is experiencing shock and disbelief. Perhaps she feels numb or things don't seem to make sense. "How can this be happening to me?" she asks, or "I can't believe this!" she exclaims. These feelings are important; they serve to protect you from overwhelming feelings and circumstances. To fully comprehend a tragedy or loss in a short period of time would be too much for your psyche to take in.

Alert

Denial allows the newly diagnosed person to take a healthy timeout and to avoid feeling overwhelmed by his change in circumstances, but it shouldn't prevent him from making decisions regarding his care. If you've been prescribed one of the disease-modifying drugs by your neurologist, it is important to begin treatment early. Taking a proactive stance will play an important role in your treatment.

Anger

Anger often creeps in once you're feeling a little less vulnerable and have gotten on with the task of living. Most people are conditioned to believe that anger is unhealthy, but it is an important part of the grieving process. It is part of your emotional management.

What you're feeling when you're in the angry stage may not always be logical. You may be angry at yourself for not preventing the disease somehow; you might be angry at your doctor for telling you in the first place, or angry at your spouse for not being more supportive. But anger is a necessary stage in the healing process, and the best thing you can do is find healthy ways to express it. Consider speaking to a therapist or a clergyman—someone who will allow you to feel safe expressing your anger or bewilderment. Activities such as gardening, walking, or swimming will help you to externalize your feelings. It's okay to scream into your pillow, too.

Just as denial provides you with an opportunity to disconnect, anger allows you the opportunity to reconnect with your feelings and your sense of self. Let's face it—you have been assigned a task you neither expected nor asked for. The life you had envisioned has been irrevocably changed without any sense of fairness. That certainly gives you reason to be angry, and it's important to express it. But don't confuse anger with helplessness. Once you have dealt with your emotions (which can be a long process) you will grab the reins again and learn to propel those emotions in a healthy and constructive way.

Bargaining

Bargaining is the process of trying to avoid painful situations by saying, "If only . . ." It is also a process of magical thinking—wishing to go back in time and somehow recreate circumstances that would have resulted in a different outcome. People diagnosed with MS often wonder if there was something they did to create the condition in their lives, or wonder if there was something they could have done to prevent it. The answer to that question is "no." There is no indication that lifestyle choices had any bearing on your diagnosis.

In the bargaining stage, you may also ask a higher power for reassurances. You may request that no other tragedies visit your family or that no other illnesses are sent your way, or assume that having been diagnosed with MS, you've somehow filled your lifetime quota for difficulty. Living in uncertainty is part of the human condition and people know intuitively that no such reassurances can be granted. But bargaining helps you get from one place to another, allowing you to feel that somehow, you can restore order to the chaotic circumstances in your life.

Part of dealing with MS is understanding that on some level, you are no longer completely in control of your own life. Part of the journey you will take in accepting the disease is learning how to balance what you can't control with what you can control. Treatment options, attitude, lifestyle choices—these things will always remain in your court.

 Essential

> MS does not have the power to steal your dreams, compromise your goals, or sabotage your life. The essence of who you are is not for sale. In the bargaining process, understand that life is unpredictable for everyone, but that most people, even in the worst possible circumstances, have learned to bring order to the chaos and empower themselves through the choices they make.

Depression

In the depression stage, grief moves into your life on a deeper level. The difficult feelings you tried to stave off with anger or bargaining have come to roost. People who experience depression often withdraw from life for a time, feel lethargic, or devoid of feeling.

Feeling depressed after sustaining a loss or adjusting to difficult life circumstances is normal. Sometimes you have to let the normal depression that comes with grief have its place in your life by acknowledging it and working through it.

Alert

> Sadness is what you feel at certain times in your life, but it is important to distinguish between sadness and clinical depression, which is depression that doesn't go away or is seriously compromising the quality of your life. Finding a therapist to support you and help you deal with your emotions is a wise choice.

Acceptance

Acceptance doesn't mean that suddenly you're okay with what has happened in your life. (You might never feel "okay" about being diagnosed with a chronic illness.) Acceptance means that you've grasped the reality of your situation and you're ready to incorporate that reality into your life. You may feel ready to reinvest in your life again and expend less energy on your loss.

While it is important to grieve and sort out your feelings, it is also important to keep a healthy perspective. MS is an unpredictable disease; science cannot yet predict its course in any individual. Advances in research and treatment give you good reasons to be hopeful and confident about your future. Armed with knowledge, support, and a proactive plan, you too, will find a way to incorporate MS into your life.

Make a Plan

Along with healthy grieving, coming up with a proactive plan for your life is another important step. Part of your plan should be targeting a disease-modifying therapy with your neurologist, deciding whom you want to share your news with, devising a plan for healthy living, and breaking down the bigger tasks—such as insurance issues or family roles—into manageable steps. Here are some tasks to consider:

Check In

Make another appointment with your neurologist. It's very likely that your last appointment with her was a blur, especially if you were diagnosed during the appointment. Since then, you've probably composed a list of questions and concerns that you'd like to address. If you haven't been prescribed a DMT, this would be a good time to do so.

Make Decisions

Decide whom you'd like to share your news with, whether it's your spouse or others you are close to. It isn't imperative right now to tell your employer or acquaintances.

Take Care

Try to incorporate a healthy diet and exercise into your life. Along with the obvious benefits, it will give you a sense of control and empowerment.

Do Some Research

Log on to *www.nationalmssociety.org* to find your local chapter of the National MS Society. Knowledge is power! It also decreases fear. The NMSS is an important resource for helping you to understand and cope with the disease. It can also provide information regarding insurance, social security, and other practical matters.

Find Support

Create a support network composed of family, friends, and health care professionals. While those closest to you can be counted on to help you sort through your feelings and manage the home front, health care professionals can guide you in making important decisions about your treatment and care. Some of the key players are your neurologist, rehabilitation professionals, and mental health counselors. Support groups can also be helpful (more on the support team in Chapter 19).

Address Your Fears

It's normal to have fears and apprehensions when diagnosed with a chronic illness, but it's good to pull them out from their hiding place to see how they're affecting you. Some people who are diagnosed with MS worry about:

- Losing a sense of who they are in the world.
- Becoming dependent on those they love.
- The people who depend on them.
- Their finances and other practical issues.
- Becoming disabled.

- Others viewing them differently if they tell them about the diagnosis.

With all of the advances in the last decade, more and more people with MS are able to face their concerns and fears with a sense of hope and optimism. These days, people with MS are a viable force in the workplace and continue to contribute to their families and the community at large. Starting treatment early and being proactive about your condition will help alleviate many of your concerns.

Educating yourself will be helpful in educating others about your disease. One expression you'll hear quite often is "But you look so good!" (Everyone with MS has heard that at least once.) That's because MS isn't a readily noticeable disease. Most people with MS (especially in the early stages) do look good. This misconception can be a problem, especially when others are making demands on your time, not realizing that just because you look well, it doesn't necessarily mean you feel well. Sharing some facts with those folks who don't understand MS can go a long way in changing the expectations and perceptions of others.

Essential

Having a strategy to address your fears is the number-one way to lessen them. Doing careful financial planning, readdressing your roles at work and home, and utilizing time management strategies are all choices that will empower you. It often takes time to figure out how your MS is going to behave, and once you do, it may be easier to plan your days and weeks accordingly.

Defining a Positive Outlook

People who deal with chronic illnesses are often told by well-meaning others to "Cheer up and look at the bright side!" or they're told that adopting a sunny and positive attitude is imperative to their health. While their advice isn't completely misguided, those with chronic illnesses sometimes feel as if they are being asked to hide their feelings and keep a smile on their face. The truth is that dealing with a chronic illness is a balance—a balance between being proactive and optimistic while still allowing yourself the luxury of feeling angry, tired, frustrated, or anxious from time to time. You don't have to be a hero.

Having said that, a positive outlook can go a long way. Learning to accept change with a sense of hope will be a tremendous asset to you. The connection between mind and body is well established. A positive outlook has many health benefits, including fewer illnesses and reduced stress.

 Alert

Flexibility is one of the most important tools in your MS toolbox. Since your symptoms may vary from day to day or month to month, being willing and able to change direction during the day will help you manage. Moving a lunch date to an air conditioned restaurant, rescheduling an outing for another day, even adopting a more flexible work schedule are examples of how you can build flexibility into your life.

One thing you will hear quite a bit on your journey to acceptance is "Don't focus on what you can't do, focus on what you can do." This is a good way to define a positive outlook; it's a glass-half-full strategy and is meant to help you focus on what is possible.

Reach Out for Support

You may feel alone and isolated with your thoughts after your diagnosis or even during a relapse. It's important to break the ice with your family members or friends and talk about your feelings. Don't keep your feelings bottled up or minimized. Requesting reassurance and emotional support from others can help relieve your tension. There are other ways to find support.

Therapy

It's great to be able to rely on friends and family members, but building a strong support network outside of the circle of our loved ones is also important. Having an unbiased and neutral ear is good for you; it offers you the opportunity to speak with a trained professional who is equipped to guide you through the ups and downs of MS.

Community Outreach Services

These services aid people in developing their personal capacity and potential. Many community service organizations offer programs on wellness, education enrichment, and self-development.

Support

Talking to others who know exactly where you're coming from is not only comforting, it's empowering. Others who have trodden the same path will have great ideas and resources to share and can also offer inspiration.

Get comfortable asking for help. You may be surprised to learn that people like to give. Be specific about your needs, whether it's help with your kids and the housework or just a shoulder to lean on.

Keeping Perspective

You don't want to let MS become the main focus of your life, although it's easy to understand how it happens. Dealing with an illness can make you feel trapped in an endless cycle of medical appointments, treatments, and self-analysis. It's important not to fall into that trap. Reminding yourself that MS is only a part of your life can help you keep things in perspective. Keep up with your friends, your favorite activities, and your hobbies.

Putting things in perspective requires you to assess your self-esteem. If you measure life events with MS as your backdrop, you are bound to feel challenged and depressed. It's important to feel good about who you are and where you are in life. What do the words "good enough" mean to you? Can you accept yourself just as you are? Can you create a space in your life that brings you happiness and joy—a reality that exists outside of MS?

See yourself as a victor, not a victim. It may help to see MS as a challenge rather than something to defeat.

Keep an MS-free zone in your life. How often do you talk about it during the day? Does it dominate your conversations with your family? If you feel it is taking more of your time and energy than you would like it to, then it may be time to start defining your boundaries. Create a time during the week when you can talk about how you're feeling with your family members or friends and resolve not to discuss MS the rest of the time. This way, you are creating a space where you can enjoy conversations with your loved ones without reverting to topics on your health.

Learning to cope with an MS diagnosis takes time. Initially, your world will feel turned upside down, so allow yourself time to grieve before picking up the reins and wrestling control. Finding and accepting support, learning as much as you can about MS, and coming up with a plan will go a long way in helping you to come to a place of acceptance. Remember that this is a process, and it will likely take some time before you get there.

CHAPTER 5

Creating an MS Management Team

FINDING THE RIGHT doctors and specialists to work with you can be a little tricky, depending on where you live and what type of health care plan you have. Not only do you want to form a team that has experience with MS, but you're also looking for the right fit—people you feel comfortable establishing a long-term relationship with. Since MS is a complex disease, you are likely to seek the expertise and advice of a range of health care professionals. Knowing who to call and how to coordinate these professionals will help you optimize your care.

Finding the Right Doctor and Specialists

Your family physician may have referred you to a neurologist for diagnosis, or he may have made the diagnosis himself. While your GP is an invaluable member of your team, it's best to see a neurologist for your long-term care, preferably one that specializes in MS. An MS specialist is armed with the latest research and studies, and understands the various options for drug treatment and symptom management.

Primary Care Physicians

Primary care physicians generally include internists, family practitioners, and pediatricians. Your primary care doctor will keep an eye on your general health and routine care; if seeing an MS specialist on a regular basis isn't possible, he can also carry out the plan decided on by you and your specialist. Not every illness or problem you encounter with your health will be MS-related; you still need a primary care physician to manage your other health needs. Your primary care physician is also a good resource; he may be able to refer you to other specialists in your area.

⌐ Essential

In your life before MS, when you only saw your doctor once or twice a year, it might not have made a difference to you whether you liked her bedside manner or her office was in a convenient location. But, as you may be spending more time with her, if you don't feel comfortable with your doctor, now is the time to find someone who better suits your needs.

If you are not able to see an MS specialist or a neurologist on a routine basis because of insurance issues or geography, make sure your primary care physician is comfortable being a player on your MS team. He will be consulting with your specialist from time to time and will also be responsible for carrying out the plan that you and your specialist determine is the best one for you.

Neurologist

A general neurologist has experience in caring for people with neurological disorders, such as Parkinson's disease, epilepsy, and strokes. She may or may not have a lot of experience and training with MS, so it's important to check.

Your health care plan may not provide you with the luxury of choosing your neurologist, so you might want to consider paying out of pocket to see a specialist once or twice a year, even if you have to travel a long distance to do so. It's hard to put a price tag on the peace of mind you'll feel.

Whether you see a general neurologist or a specialist (or whether your primary care physician is managing your care, in coordination with a neurologist), you want to feel confident that you are getting the best medical treatment available to you. Research into MS is constantly evolving, so finding a doctor who's on top of the most recent studies is important. Asking the physician about his experience with MS should be on the top of your checklist when looking for a good doctor.

Fact

A recent survey revealed that 63 percent of the respondents were diagnosed by a general neurologist. MS specialists diagnosed 28 percent, and 9 percent received a diagnosis from an assortment of other medical practitioners, including ophthalmologists, neurosurgeons, radiologists, and family doctors.

Your Doctor's Credentials

So, you've found a doctor you feel comfortable with and who has the necessary experience in treating your condition. Now it's time to check out your doctor's credentials. Experts say that people spend more time researching the purchase of their next car than they do their doctor's qualifications, so don't feel foolish investing your time in this important endeavor. The American Medical Association recommends that you research the following credentials:

- **Is your doctor board certified?** A doctor who is board certified has taken several extra years of specialty training and has passed a rigorous board examination. Some boards require continuing education and periodic recertification.
- **What is your doctor's academic history?** It's important to know your doctor's area of specialization and subspecialization— the areas in which a doctor has received between three to seven years of additional training beyond medical school.
- **What hospital is your doctor affiliated with?** Information about her affiliations will tell you if a doctor has a relationship with a particular hospital. Is this a hospital that is convenient for you? Is it a hospital that you trust and feel comfortable going to?

In addition to training and experience, what else are you looking for in a specialist?

Likability Factor

Let's face it—you're going to be sharing a lot with your specialist, so it's important to feel comfortable with her. Not all great doctors have great bedside manners, so you'll want to figure out what characteristics are most important to you. Are you looking for warm and fuzzy or the gentle, bookish type? Do you want an eager doctor fresh out of medical school or one who's been in practice for years?

Communication Factor

Does your specialist answer your questions fully and treat you with compassion and respect? Determine whether the doctor welcomes or resists your questions. A doctor should be willing to listen to all of your concerns, be open to your ideas, and be candid yet caring.

Convenience Factor

Make sure you inquire about the doctor's office hours. You'll also want to know how responsive she will be to your phone calls and inquiries as well as the average wait time for appointments. Note the location and accessibility of the office. You can find the answers to these questions by calling and speaking to a member of her staff—a nurse, an assistant, or a receptionist.

Question

Where do I find an MS specialist?
If your doctor or insurance company cannot help you locate an MS specialist, there are many resources available to help you. The NMSS, which stresses the importance of finding competent neurologists, has a service to help people find a doctor in their area. You can also solicit recommendations from friends or relatives or you can check with area hospitals for a referral. Your county medical society and medical insurance company may also be able to help. Call 1-800-FIGHT-MS for more information.

Teamwork Factor

Ask your neurologist if she is comfortable with calling on the expertise of other doctors in the course of your care. You may need to utilize the skills of other doctors and specialists, such as social workers, psychologists, urologists, and physical therapists. Your neurologist will likely coordinate your care with these specialists.

Routine Care with a Neurologist

Once you've established a diagnosis, selected a neurologist, and decided on a course of treatment, you'll establish a pattern of routine care. Most MS specialists see their patients two times per year, but that number can vary depending on your status. During your visits, your doctor will monitor disease progression and help you get a handle on your symptoms. Some MS specialists request an MRI intermittently to keep an eye on your lesion load and gauge the effectiveness of your treatment.

Fact

> As of 2003, individuals in all states were given the right to request and inspect their medical records under a new federal health privacy regulation. Review your medical records carefully to ensure that the information is correct. Any errors you note should be directed to your physician.

Not only have you picked a doctor, you've also established a member of your team to manage your health. You both have a role to play. What can you do to optimize your visits and make them easy for you both? Preparing for your appointment ahead of time will make the visit much more productive.

- **Bring along your journal.** It's important to keep track of your symptoms, their severity, and other worries or concerns so you can share them with your doctor. Prioritize your biggest concerns to make the most of the time you have.
- **Don't forget your medical records.** This is especially important during your first visit. Your records might include MRI scans, test results, and records from your previous doctors.
- **Bring a list of your medications.** If you're taking an over-the-counter medication or prescription medication (including vitamins, herbs, and supplements), be sure to let your doctor know the exact dosage and how many times a day you take them.
- **Decide what you'd like to get out of the appointment ahead of time.** If you have six issues you'd like to discuss, you may only have time to address three. Consider making another appointment or booking a double appointment if you feel you need more time.
- **Bring along an appointment buddy.** Having a friend or family member come with you will help you to remember important information from your visit. They can take notes for you, or just act as a "second ear" during your appointment.

Beyond routine visits, you may also call your specialist when you are experiencing an exacerbation (typically a new symptom that lasts more than twenty-four hours), or when you have questions or concerns about your treatment, or you feel you need to enlist the services of another specialist (a urologist or psychologist, for example).

The Team Approach

Because MS can present a myriad of symptoms, the team approach has become an effective and efficient way to provide comprehensive care. Your neurologist will be an invaluable tool in helping you to identify your needs. Not everyone with MS has the same type of doctors or health care specialists. What physicians you see will depend on what your symptoms are. A person who has bladder issues, for example, will see a urologist, while someone who is experiencing problems with muscle weakness will see a rehabilitation specialist. Who are the other key players in treating MS?

 Alert

> Contrary to popular belief, the time you spend with your physician has gotten longer, not shorter, in the past fifteen years. A 2002 study showed the average time spent with a doctor is 18.4 minutes, up by almost three minutes compared to 1989. Despite this, you may not always have enough time to address all of your concerns. Scheduling a double appointment when you've got a lot of things you'd like to discuss is a good idea.

Your Doctor's Staff

Most doctors' offices are staffed with receptionists, nurses, and, more often than not, a physician's assistant (PA). Getting to know the receptionist is a good idea; she may be able to schedule a last-minute appointment for you on a particularly busy day or give you the real lowdown on how long it might take for the doctor to call you back.

Nurses are an invaluable part of the doctor's staff. Whether by phone or in the office, nurses often take on the role of supporter, and are there to answer your questions, address your concerns, and provide education. Nurses who specialize in MS are particularly helpful, as they are well educated in the disease process and treatment management. Busy doctors often rely on them to play a key role in the care of patients.

Some neurology offices and MS centers employ PAs, though you're more likely to come across one in your primary care office. A PA is a licensed health professional who practices medicine under the supervision of a physician. The scope of their work is regulated by the state they are licensed in, but almost all PAs can visit with patients, order lab tests, perform physical exams, and in some cases, make a diagnosis. In general, they perform 80 percent of the tasks that doctors perform. PAs assist neurologists in busy offices, most often for routine neurological exams. If your doctor employs a PA and you'd prefer to see your neurologist, let the receptionist know when you call to schedule an appointment.

Fact

A study conducted in the United Kingdom underscored the importance of having an MS-specialized nurse as a staff member in a specialist's office. Patients reported an increased benefit to their knowledge, mood, and ability to cope with the disease. A study in the United States showed that certified MS nurses were rated better than doctors on interpersonal skills, technical-care skills, and giving information.

Urologists

Eighty percent of people diagnosed with MS have trouble with their bladder during the course of the disease. Problems range from urinary frequency to difficulty emptying the bladder. A urologist will help you to identify the cause of the problems in your urinary tract and offer treatment.

Rehabilitation Specialists

The goal of rehabilitation is to keep people with MS productive and independent, with an emphasis on quality of life. These specialists provide services that restore function, improve mobility, and relieve pain. A rehabilitation program is designed to meet the needs of the individual patient depending on the type and severity of symptoms. Your physician (most likely your neurologist) will assist you in deciding what services you need and will refer you to the appropriate specialist.

Physical Therapist (PT)

A physical therapist's job is to build strength, flexibility, and spirit. The PT will evaluate your current level of strength, mobility, posture, and balance and will help you compensate for any changes brought about by MS. The PT can help with balance problems, weakness, fatigue, pain, and lack of coordination.

Occupational Therapist (OT)

Occupational therapy can be very beneficial if your symptoms are preventing you from performing the tasks of everyday life or involve weakness, lack of coordination, or tremor of the arms. OTs can provide assessment and treatment for in-home adaptations such as cooking, eating, driving, and handwriting. They can also be invaluable in helping you to adapt your workplace environment to suit your needs.

Vocational Rehabilitation Specialist

A vocational rehabilitation specialist can help people with MS remove barriers that may prevent them from having a satisfying career. Or, if a change of scenery in the workplace is needed, a specialist can pull available resources together to assist in helping to make career choices. A counselor can assist by being an advocate in employment situations, giving vocational testing to target new jobs or careers, and also researching disability benefits offered through an employer. They're a good source of advice when deciding whether or not to disclose your condition to an employer.

Essential

Experts say people keep better financial, car, and pet records than they do medical records and too often rely on their doctors to do this. Keeping and reading your own medical records will help to avoid medical errors or mishaps. You'll have them handy for the emergency room or visits to a specialist.

Speech Pathologist

Speech-language pathologists, sometimes called speech therapists, assess, diagnose, treat, and help to prevent speech, language, fluency, cognitive-communication, voice, swallowing, and other related disorders. People with MS see a speech pathologist when they are experiencing problems with swallowing or speech. In addition, some speech pathologists evaluate and treat cognitive difficulties.

Audiologist

Sometimes people with MS develop hearing or balance problems. Some people also deal with tinnitus, which causes a ringing sound in the inner ear. An audiologist, who is trained to handle hearing and balance problems, can assess, diagnose, and treat these symptoms. Your primary care physician or neurologist can refer you to an audiologist for treatment.

Registered Dietician

Registered dieticians provide nutritional counseling through diet management to promote good nutrition. They are available to assess your nutritional needs and recommend changes in your diet, since good nutrition is vital to your well-being.

Mental Health Counselors

Counselors or therapists provide a variety of services to people with MS and are invaluable when it comes to caring for your emotional health. Services range from teaching stress-management skills to providing psychiatric medications or coordinating community resources. Counselors and therapists can be found in medical clinics, mental health centers, or in private practice.

Social Worker

Social workers give personal support to people with MS by providing referrals for short- and long term counseling and recommending resources for both community and national agencies that support people with MS. In addition, they can offer information about home-care assistance and assistive devices as well as providing financial information such as details about social security disability and Medicaid.

Psychiatrist

Psychiatrists are medical physicians who specialize in the diagnosis, treatment, and prevention of mental illnesses. They also prescribe medication that helps manage mental health conditions such as depression or anxiety. In most states, psychiatrists are the only mental health professionals who can write a prescription, so you may be referred to one by a social worker, psychologist, or other mental health professional.

Clinical Psychologist

Clinical psychologists help people with MS cope with the interpersonal, emotional, and cognitive aspects of the disease by offering individual and group counseling and by evaluating psychological and emotional problems. They can also provide neuropsychological testing to help pinpoint areas of cognitive difficulty, such as problems with memory.

Neuropsychologist

Neuropsychologists are clinical psychologists who specialize in memory, problem-solving, and other cognitive problems and can also diagnose MS. Neuropsychologists may also offer cognitive rehabilitation exercises to improve memory, attention, information processing, and reasoning.

Other Types of Counselors

If you've ever looked up "therapist" or "counselor" in your yellow pages, you may have noticed the multitude of choices, including licensed and unlicensed therapists along with personal, family, and marriage counselors. In addition to getting referrals from family members or health professionals, you must also identify your needs. Do you simply want someone to talk to, or do you need help with family or marriage issues? Finding a therapist who has experience with chronic illnesses should be at the top of your list. They understand the impact that an illness can have on families and individuals.

Coordinating Your Team

Don't let all the various health care professionals listed here overwhelm you. Very few people with MS will need all of them, and most will need only a few. The important thing to remember is that you are the team captain. Even though it can be difficult to keep track of all the players, these professionals are there to help you treat and cope with MS.

Even with the best of intentions, today's health care professionals can be so overburdened with insurance regulations, heavy patient loads and administrative duties that things can "fall through the cracks." It's up to you to make sure they don't. Following are a few ideas to keep the scorecard straight.

Be a Good Record Keeper

Keep a notebook and use it specifically for medical information, preferably one with a calendar. A good daily planner serves several different functions and has various options to choose from including a calendar, an address book, and a space to write notes in for specific days. List all of the members of your health care team. Use the calendar to keep track of appointments and use the daily notebook section to record the outcome of the appointment so it is at your fingertips when you need to refer to it. Have a good filing cabinet and a system set up to file insurance papers, medical records, and other important paperwork.

Alert

If you are organizationally challenged, ask a family member or a social worker to help you set up a functional system for record keeping. Not having to dig through a pile of papers every time you need something will save you time and reduce your stress load. Even those who live without a chronic illness have a hard time with hills of paperwork to sift through. Keeping ahead of the game will allow you more time to do those things that are not MS-related.

Plan Carefully

Keeping track of your appointments is essential. It is also important to prioritize your appointments and tasks. For example, you should check with your insurance carrier before making an appointment with a neuropsychologist to make sure you're covered.

Essential

Many people aren't aware that care managers are available—a relatively new professional who helps plan and organize care for people with illnesses or disabilities. These professionals can coordinate care with community services, such as arranging for meals, finding and hiring needed help, finding a lawyer, or even finding someone to mow the lawn.

Don't Assume Anything

It is important that your doctors communicate among themselves, but don't assume they do. Make sure each clinician makes a copy of all your records and reports and sends them to the other members of your health care team. Of course, you'll want a copy for your own records. Your primary care physician or your neurologist (whomever you've selected) will be the coordinator of these services. Make sure that he receives copies of your records from your other clinicians and that he's always kept in the loop.

Communicate

In addition to helping your doctors communicate with each other, you also need to be a good communicator. Let each clinician know about other recent appointments you've had or if your medications have recently changed.

Comprehensive MS Treatment Centers

Not everyone lives near an MS center, but if you do, you may want to consider using one for your care. MS centers provide a range of specialists under one roof so you don't have to be referred to other specialists for specific issues.

MS centers offer convenience, combining onsite physical, occupational, and behavioral therapy, often with state-of-the-art medical treatment to manage MS and its associated symptoms in one building. You don't have to worry about running from appointment to appointment. MS centers are likely to offer diagnostic services, a comprehensive list of doctors and specialists, comprehensive treatment, and opportunities for education.

Many MS centers participate in MS clinical research trials. Patients at these centers are often able to take advantage of new treatments before they are available elsewhere. You can find the MS center nearest to you by contacting the Consortium of MS Centers (*www.mscare.org*) or by contacting the NMSS at 1-800-FIGHT-MS or *www.national mssociety.org*.

Establish a Relationship with Your Health Care Team

In addition to the suggestions given above for optimizing your visits with your neurologist, there are other things you can do to encourage a healthy and productive relationship with all of your health team members. Establishing a trusting relationship with your doctor is essential if you are to feel a sense of self-empowerment and control over your life.

Be an Effective Patient

Being involved in your own care largely depends on your own personal style. Some people want to take a more active role in their health care and have clear ideas about their treatments. Others may be more inclined to look to their doctors for guidance. Whatever your style, being effective means participating. Ask questions and, time permitting, bring in research or studies that interest you. It's important to feel that you are contributing to the care you are receiving.

Have Realistic Expectations

While your doctor should listen to your questions and concerns, be accessible in emergencies, and return your calls, he isn't your mother or your best friend. Have realistic expectations about his involvement in your care.

Speak Up

Don't hesitate to tell your doctor if you're dissatisfied and give him an opportunity to correct the problem. For example, you could say, "I have concerns as to why you are suggesting this approach." Be concerned, but not accusatory.

Clarify

At the end of the appointment, ask your doctor to clarify anything about your treatment that you don't understand. It's also a good idea to summarize what he's discussed with you to make sure you've heard him correctly. Ask your doctor to write down anything you may have trouble remembering.

Your relationship with your doctors is like any partnership—communication is the key. Ideally, your neurologist or primary care physician should provide most of your care. If specialty care is needed, your doctor's knowledge about your health history will make it easier to coordinate your care with specialists who are likely to meet your needs.

CHAPTER 6

The Treatment of MS

LIKE THE DISEASE itself, treating MS is multifaceted. Strategies include modifying the disease course, treating exacerbations, and managing symptoms. Just as no two people with MS are alike, no two treatment plans are the same. Your care will largely depend on your symptoms and disease type. The first line of defense in treating MS is deciding you are going to take charge. Be determined to meet each and every challenge presented to you with a sense of spunk and determination.

Early Treatment Makes a Difference

As noted in an earlier chapter, starting treatment early is one of the most important factors in managing MS. Researchers have discovered that the disease process may begin well before any obvious symptoms arise, allowing damage to occur in the brain and spinal cord. The earlier you begin treatment, the better your chances of minimizing nerve damage and halting progression.

Since many people who are diagnosed with MS have relapsing-remitting disease, they often question whether starting one of the disease-modifying therapies (DMTs) immediately is right for them. They may be feeling good at the moment and have their symptoms under control. They may also hesitate to begin treatment because it is a long-term commitment that must be monitored by a health care provider; it has an impact on their lives. However, evidence supports the need for early treatment:

- Experts agree that damage to the CNS occurs very early in the disease process, even before symptoms appear.
- Treatments may shorten the length and decrease the severity of exacerbations.
- Treatments may also modify the disease course, slowing the advance of MS.
- Treatments can extend remissions, or the period of time between exacerbations.

The goal of treatment, then, is to slow irreversible damage by preventing the inflammatory process that can lead to demyelination and axon damage. Therapy generally isn't a cure, but it's a good line of defense in helping you to stay as healthy as possible for as long as possible.

Fact

A clinically isolated episode may be monofocal, in which symptoms present at a single site in the central nervous system, or multifocal, in which multiple sites exhibit symptoms. So you might experience a lone symptom, such as optic neuritis, or several symptoms at once, such as sensory symptoms and muscle weakness.

Starting a DMT Before a Definite Diagnosis

Deciding whether to start a DMT before you've received a definite MS diagnosis is a decision that you and your physician can explore together. People who have experienced a clinically isolated syndrome (CIS: one neurological episode, lasting at least twenty-four hours and caused by inflammation in the CNS) may or may not go on to develop MS. However, studies show that those presenting with certain signs or symptoms have a greater chance of developing MS. If a CIS is accompanied by evidence of MS-type lesions on an MRI, the likelihood of having a second neurological episode is greater.

Three large-scale clinical trials have been conducted to determine whether early treatment following a clinically isolated syndrome can delay a second clinical event. The studies involved the use of Avonex, Betaseron, and Rebif (three of the DMTs used in MS) and results indicated that the drugs significantly delayed the onset of a second neurological episode. MRI findings also showed that the brain lesion volume in the patients studied was reduced. It is important to discuss these studies with your doctor and decide which course of action is right for you.

Alert

Deciding which drug to take is also a lifestyle choice. One drug, for example, must be injected daily, while another is injected once per week. Carefully considering your schedule and preferences may help you to decide which drug is best for you. Knowing that the drugs have similar effectiveness may make it easier for you to choose.

The Disease-Modifying Therapies

There are currently six FDA-approved medications on the market that modify the course of MS. These drugs are known as immuno-modulating medications and their job is to alter the activity of the immune system. The most important goal is to find a treatment you can use comfortably and consistently. The pharmaceutical companies that manufacture and market the MS disease-modifying drugs offer various types of support to their customers. They may also provide some financial assistance for qualifying individuals without prescription drug coverage. It is important to contact your health insurance provider to discuss your coverage before filling a prescription. Most people rely on some type of insurance or financial support, as these drugs are expensive.

As with any drug you are considering, it is important to discuss your options with your physician. If you are planning to get pregnant, are nursing, or have a history of depression or liver problems, you should let your doctor know before starting a DMT. In fact, make a list of any health concerns you have.

Choosing a treatment that works best for you is an important part of taking control of the disease. There are several factors to weigh when considering a drug. For example, you should list the possible side effects from the drug and read the current studies on the drug's performance. You should also read the safety information on any drugs prescribed and be comfortable with the risks involved.

Your goal in choosing a therapy is to find one that is effective, but you also want to choose one that works well with your lifestyle and that you can stick with. Right now, the DMTs are your best line of defense.

Essential

There's a lot to tackle when deciding which disease-modifying therapy is best for you. There are websites, books, pamphlets, and organizations that can arm you with information. Just be sure to use trusted resources, such as the National MS Society. Of course, your physician is one of your most trusted team members, so be sure to address your questions to him or other members of your health care team.

Injectable Immunomodulating Medications

Avonex, Betaseron, Copaxone, and Rebif are the four injectable immunomodulating medications available for the treatment of MS. There are two classes of these drugs:

- Interferons (IFNs)
- Glatiramer acetate (copolymer-1)

Both drug classes have been shown to slow down the disease process and reduce the risk of future attacks or exacerbations.

The Interferons

The interferons are proteins produced naturally by the body that fight viral infections and help regulate the immune system. The interferon medications for MS are made up of the same amino acids as the interferon found in the body but they are manufactured using biotechnology. No one is sure exactly how they work, but it is believed that they help regulate the body's immune response against myelin. Researchers are studying the interferons to understand how they work. It is hoped the answers to their questions will assist them in developing new treatments.

All three interferons are approved for use in relapsing-remitting MS.

Avonex (interferon beta-1a)

Avonex is a product of the Biogen Idec pharmaceutical company and is a form of interferon beta. This drug is approved for the relapsing-remitting form of MS and has also been approved for use by individuals who have had a clinically isolated syndrome. The goal of Avonex therapy is to slow the natural progression of disability and reduce exacerbations. Avonex is administered once a week through intramuscular injections, which means the drug must be injected directly into the muscle—usually the thigh muscle or the muscles in the upper arm.

As with any prescription medication, side effects can occur. Keep in mind that many of the side effects subside over time.

- Flu-like symptoms (particularly at the start of treatment)
- Muscle aches
- Fever
- Chills
- Weakness
- Depression

Anyone who has a history of depression should tell their doctors before starting Avonex or any of the interferon drugs, as they may worsen depression in some people.

Betaseron (interferon beta-1b)

Betaseron, made by Bayer HealthCare was, the first drug shown to be effective in the treatment of relapsing-remitting MS. Like Avonex, it is an interferon, though with a slightly different chemical makeup. When compared to the outcome of those taking a placebo in a two-year study, results showed that Betaseron reduced the number and severity of exacerbations along with a reduction in the number of brain lesions. It has also been approved to treat people with CIS and has been shown to delay the onset of MS.

Betaseron is administered every other day by subcutaneous injection, which means under the skin and not in a muscle. A side effect of Betaseron is a reaction at the injection site, but this too may subside over time. It is important to rotate injection sites each time you administer the drug. Other side effects include:

- Flu-like symptoms (particularly at the beginning of treatment)
- Depression

Rebif (interferon beta-1a)

Rebif (Pfizer, EMD, Serono) has been shown to reduce the number and severity of exacerbations, reduce new or active lesions on MRI, and slow the progression of disability. It has not been approved by the FDA for use in individuals with CIS, but has demonstrated its ability to delay the onset of MS in people with CIS.

Rebif is administered three times a week by subcutaneous injection and is available in prefilled syringes.

Common side effects include:

- Flu-like symptoms (particularly at the start of treatment)
- Injection-site reactions
- Depression

Glatiramer Acetate (copolymer-1)

The second class of immunomodulating drugs is glatiramer acetate. Copaxone, made by Teva Neuroscience, is a noninterferon drug, which means it has a different line of defense than Rebif, Avonex, and Betaseron. The interferons seem to prevent confused cells from crossing the blood-brain barrier to attack myelin, while glatiramer acetate seems to block myelin-damaging T cells by serving as a decoy. As with the interferon drugs, studies have shown that Copaxone has beneficial effects on exacerbations, MRI lesions, and disability. It is approved by the FDA to treat relapsing-remitting MS.

Copaxone is administered daily by subcutaneous injection. Side effects include:

- Injection-site reactions
- In some people, chest tightness, shortness of breath, and flushing immediately after administering a shot, but these problems resolve within fifteen minutes without further problems

Infusion Treatments

Some MS medications are infusion treatments, which means that the medication is a liquid that is administered directly into the bloodstream through a vein in your arm.

Infusion treatments are typically given in several different settings: a specially equipped doctor's office, an infusion center, or a hospital. Your vital signs will be recorded before, during, and after the medication is administered, and you will be asked to watch for any type of allergic reaction such as hives, chills, itching, or rash. Allergic reactions are rare but can occur any time after the treatment is administered, most often within several hours after an infusion.

Fact

The DMTs have been found to reduce the relapse rate in people with MS by 30 percent. They do not reverse the effects and symptoms of MS that have already developed or become permanent before the treatment is started. The treatments won't make you feel better, but may be your best line of defense against future relapses.

Immunosuppressants

Immunosuppressants are medications that shut down the body's immune system. These drugs are primarily used to treat cancer and are used in individuals with MS in whom the disease is worsening and first-line drug therapies, such as the interferons or Copaxone, have not been effective.

Novantrone (mitoxantrone)

Novantrone (EMD Serono) was approved more than a decade ago to fight certain types of cancer. In 2000, the FDA approved the use of Novantrone to treat people with relapsing-remitting MS that is worsening as well as for people with progressive-relapsing or secondary progressive MS. The recommended treatment schedule for use in MS is far less frequent than it is for cancer treatment, and thus the side effects are more manageable. Keep in mind that Novantrone is not intended for use as a treatment for people with primary progressive MS.

In clinical trials, Novantrone showed a reduction in the relapse rate of people with MS, as well as a reduction in the number of lesions on MRI scans and a slowing of disability progression. Novantrone is believed to work by inhibiting the immune cells that attack the CNS. It is usually administered intravenously once every three months.

Alert

Because Novantrone can damage your heart, patients are carefully monitored. Before treatment begins, your heart will be checked by your doctor using an echocardiogram or similar study. Doses of the drug are limited to eight to twelve over a two- to three-year period, and cardiac testing is recommended before each dose.

When using Novantrone, your doctor will also take blood samples to check your blood counts and liver function. If you are a woman of childbearing age, your doctor will also give you a pregnancy test before treatment begins each time. While this protocol might seem a bit overwhelming, your doctor wants to be sure that Novantrone is the best drug for you and that your heart and liver are in good working order from the get-go.

Question

What is LDN?
LDN stands for low dose naltrexone, an FDA-approved drug used for treating addiction. Over the last decade anecdotal reports have stated that LDN is effective in providing symptom relief in some people with MS. Currently, the University of California–San Francisco MS Center is conducting a study on LDN, which patient advocates helped to fund.

Other side effects of Novantrone include an increased risk for secondary acute myelogenous leukemia (rare), nausea, hair loss, and changes in the menstrual cycle.

In addition to Novantrone, other immunosuppressive drugs include methotrexate, Cytoxan (cyclophosphamide), Imuran (azathioprine) and Leustatin (cladribine). The FDA has not approved these drugs specifically for MS, but they are used sometimes in patients who do not respond to the first-line-treatment drugs for MS.

The Scoop on Tysabri

Tysabri was approved by the FDA in 2004 for relapsing forms of MS, but was then withdrawn from the market by the manufacturer (Biogen Idec) because of safety concerns. It was approved to return to the market in 2006 with a special restricted distribution program. Tysabri is the newest of the immunomodulating drugs and is not approved for people with primary progressive or secondary progressive MS.

Tysabri is administered every four weeks by intravenous infusion. It works by preventing damaging immune cells from crossing the blood-brain barrier and entering the CNS. It is usually used in cases where other MS medications have not worked. Tysabri has been proven to decrease the number of exacerbations, slow down the progression of disabling effects from MS, and reduce the number of lesions seen on MRI scans. To date, there has been no study directly comparing Tysabri to existing treatments to prove whether or not it is superior to those treatments.

While Tysabri is considered to be a very effective therapy, it is balanced by risk. In clinical trials of Tysabri, three people involved in the studies developed a rare disorder of the nervous system called progressive multifocal leukoencephalopathy (PML). PML primarily affects individuals with suppressed immune systems and is caused by a virus called the JC virus. This virus lies dormant in the immune system of most people, but in individuals who have a suppressed immune system (such as people with AIDS or those who are being treated with chemotherapy), the virus can become active and cause progressive neurological symptoms. PML is usually fatal. Two of the three people who had PML during the clinical trials of Tysabri died. One of them had been diagnosed with MS (the other had been in the trial for Crohn's disease). The FDA approved Tsyabri's re-entry into the market in 2006 after there were no additional cases of PML reported.

 Fact

The people in the MS clinical trial who developed PML were taking Tysabri in combination with Avonex, and because of this, the FDA has indicated Tsyabri's use as a monotherapy, meaning it cannot be used in combination with other disease-modifying drugs for MS.

The manufacturer, Biogen Idec, has developed a risk management plan called the TOUCH (Tysabri Outreach: Unified Commitment to Health) Prescribing Program to ensure safe use of the product. Here are the details of the plan:

- Only patients who are enrolled in the mandatory TOUCH program will be able to receive Tysabri.
- Heath care providers and their staff, infusion centers, and pharmacies must all be registered with the TOUCH program and complete an education program about the risks of Tysabri treatment.
- Before each infusion, a checklist must be completed by the patient and nurse to help track any new signs or symptoms that may require an evaluation by a physician. This ensures careful monitoring of the drug.
- Patients will be evaluated three and six months after starting Tysabri and then every six months thereafter.
- Patients with a compromised immune system or those who are taking other disease-modifying drugs for MS are not eligible for the treatment.

Based on current information, the FDA puts the risk of developing PML at 1 in 1,000. If you are considering Tysabri, it is important to balance the risks with the benefits. Keep in mind that Tysabri is indicated for people with relapsing forms of MS, meaning that some people with progressive forms of MS who still experience relapses may be candidates for Tysabri.

Common side effects of Tysabri include infusion reactions, fatigue, headaches, and joint pain. Less common (4 percent of patients) are severe allergic reactions to the drug that may cause hives/itching, chills, dizziness, chest pain, flushing, trouble breathing, and low blood pressure. People on Tysabri may be more susceptible to infections and should take measures to avoid them, including good hand-washing habits and avoiding people who are sick, when possible. Tysabri should also not be used by women who are pregnant and should be stopped for some time before trying to conceive (discuss this with your doctor). Women who are breastfeeding also should not use Tysabri.

Question

Is Tysabri associated with melanoma?
Two cases of melanoma were observed in women who began using Tysabri. Researchers have not yet established a relationship between the drug and melanoma, but they're cautioning anyone with a personal or family history of melanoma to visit a dermatologist before starting the drug.

Managing Side Effects

As of yet, the perfect drug—one that is effective without side effects—does not exist. But treatment, as you'll soon discover, is a balance, one where you must weigh the risks against the benefits. The uncertainty in predicting the course of MS means that you will have to make tough treatment decisions without any guarantees that the drug will be effective for you or that the side effects will be minimal.

As with any new venture in life, arming yourself with knowledge will help you to make a well-informed decision. Knowing what to watch for when you start a new treatment is important, but try to start the treatment without any preconceived notions of what may happen to you. Side effects vary from person to person. The woman who sits next to you at your support group may react much differently to a treatment than you do. The truth is, it's hard to know beforehand just how you will react, so the best line of defense is to be informed about potential side effects without expecting them to occur.

Fact

According to respondents from a 2007 survey, the most important aspect of a drug is its effectiveness in treating MS. Number two is affordability and number three is side effects. The survey seems to say that people with MS do not consider the side effects of a drug to have as much bearing on their willingness to include it in their treatment plan as effectiveness and affordability.

Side Effects from CRAB

CRAB is an acronym for Copaxone, Rebif, Avonex, and Betaseron—the first-line disease-modifying therapies—and those often prescribed for relapsing-remitting MS. The side effects listed for these drugs differ slightly from one to the next, but here's a list of the common side effects and suggestions on how to manage them:

Flu-like Symptoms

Interferons (Avonex, Betaseran, Rebif) may cause flu-like side effects, such as fever, chills, muscle aches, and tiredness. For many people, these side effects lessen or go away over time. If you do experience these symptoms, talk to your doctor. He may be able to recommend ways to get symptom relief, such as taking over-the-counter pain medications that help reduce pain or fever. You may also want to change the time of day you take your injection. Bedtime is a good time; you may be able to sleep through the unpleasant side effects. If you need a day to rest after your injection, make sure to clear your calendar in advance.

Fatigue

Fatigue is often a common symptom of MS, but it can also be caused by interferons. Talk to your doctor. He may have some tips to help you manage fatigue, such as exercise or medication used for fatigue. Scheduling rest time in the afternoon is also a good idea.

Injection-Site Reactions

Injection-site reactions, which may be cause by subcutaneous injections (Betaseron, Rebif, Copaxon) usually involve superficial redness, minor skin irritation, minor allergic skin reaction, and possibly infection. The best line of defense is to avoid the reactions. Try rotating the injection site and don't use the same site more than once every two weeks. Be sure to leave enough room between sites used in the same general area. Keeping an injection log may be helpful to ensure proper site rotation.

Essential

Before injecting your MS drugs, be sure to wash and rinse the site with plain soap and water and then dry it well. Do not use perfume or creams on injection-site areas, as they may cause irritation. Place a cold cloth or cool pack on the injection site before and after each injection.

Side Effects for Infusion Treatments

The side effects for infusion therapy vary but can often be controlled. Some of the reported side effects include headaches, which may be helped by over-the-counter medication. Let your doctor know if you experience any side effects.

Depression is a common side effect of MS, but mood changes—such as depression—have been noted in some people who use interferon (Avonex, Betaseron, Rebif) therapy. Talk to your doctor about any changes in your mood. Antidepressants and/or counseling may be able to help you manage.

Sometimes MS treatments can cause changes in menstruation, such as irregular bleeding, or early or late periods. Speak to a gynecologist if you experience menstruation changes that concern you.

Injection treatments may cause reactions at the injection site, such as redness, bruising and pain. Rotating the injection site, placing a cold pack on the area before and after the injection, and using cortisone cream may be helpful in reducing skin irritation from injection.

No matter which treatment you decide on, learning to integrate disease-modifying therapy into your schedule and managing its side effects are important ways to help you stay on the therapy, which is your best line of defense at the moment.

Treatment Support

It's not easy for anyone to make changes in their lives, particularly if they have to adjust their routines or if the drugs prescribed cause unpleasant side effects. At some point, you may need support—whether you're looking for help in managing side effects, you need a pep talk, or you need assistance in administering the drugs.

The Drug Companies

The companies that develop and market the various therapies for MS have a support staff to help answer your questions and address your concerns. All of the companies have toll-free numbers to call, and some have online programs that offer a variety of tools, such as sending you reminders on treatment days, offering online education seminars and twenty-four-hour-a-day nursing assistance by phone.

Besides your physician, the drug companies can play an important role in helping to make your MS treatment successful.

Betaseron

The maker of Betaseron (Bayer Health Care) offer a comprehensive online support program, as well as the B.E.T.A. program, which offers twenty-four-hour-a-day nursing support by phone. Betaseron also offers the Pathways Program, which offers free online interactive webcasts on various topics concerning MS, an online patient journal to help you manage your care, and an injection reminder calendar. Pathways is open to all people with MS and not just those taking Betaseron. To learn more, visit *www.betaseron.com* or call 1-800-788-1467.

Avonex

The maker of Avonex and Tysabri (Biogen Idec) offers a comprehensive online support program that includes educational programs, a mentoring program, a resource center, and a newsletter. A nursing services program with phone support and at-home nursing services for injection education and assistance are available to Avonex users. To learn more, visit *www.avonex.com* or *www.tysabri.com*.

Copaxone

The maker of Copaxone (Teva Neuroscience) has an online program called Shared Solutions that offers nursing support by phone, peer support, a newsletter, and educational resources including teleconferences. To learn more, visit *www.copaxone.com*.

Rebif

The makers of Rebif (EMD, Serono and Pfizer) and Novantrone (EMD Serono) have a program called MS Lifelines that offers nursing support by phone, live web events that focus on MS education and support, and other resources available on their website. To learn more, visit *www.rebif.com* or *www.novantrone.com*.

In addition to the drug companies, there are other sources of support to help you with treatment questions and concerns:

- **Your doctor and his staff.** Your doctor is your best resource for questions pertaining to your chosen therapy and its side effects. If available, an MS nurse can also provide the proper education, communication, and support to help with patient adherence to the drugs.
- **National MS Society.** The National MS Society offers brochures and online education regarding the various MS therapies. They can also help you find a support group in your area. Visit *www.nationalmssociety.org* or call 1-800-FIGHT-MS.

When choosing a DMT, the good news is that there is no shortage of help to aid you in the decision-making process. The drug companies can you give you a good overview of their DMTs, such as injection schedules, side effects, and costs. Your physician and his staff can offer valuable insight on these drugs as well, helping you to round out the picture and discover which drug may be more suited to your lifestyle.

Being Realistic about DMTs
In addition to obtaining the support you need to be consistent with your therapy, you should also have realistic expectations. The DMTs do not generally cure MS or completely prevent relapses.

Adherence to these therapies is the key to their success. Patients who are educated about a drug and receive ongoing support have the best success with their treatment plan. It's been shown that most adherence difficulties occur within the first six months of treatment, so it's important to find support if you are experiencing problems.

Recognizing Problems with DMTs
Despite all of your efforts in adhering to a therapy, at some point you and your doctor may decide a new line of defense is in order if your current medication does not appear to be effective for you. There are several reasons someone who is committed to drug

therapy may decide to switch from one treatment option to another, including a significant number of relapses, signs of disability progression, or new MRI lesions. Side effects and problematic injection-site reactions should also be discussed with your doctor, but she may be able to help you manage them.

Deciding to switch therapies is an important decision and one that must be made by both you and your physician. Although MS researchers and physicians are currently trying to come up with guidelines that will help better define the criteria for changing therapies, some of the indications listed above may be used as a marker to aid your doctor in making an informed decision.

While interferons (Avonex, Betaseron, and Rebif) and Copaxone have been shown to have beneficial effects in MS, it may take months for these drugs to produce their full therapeutic effects. What this means for you is that a poor initial response to treatment doesn't necessarily mean the treatment isn't working. Your doctor may advise you to wait at least a year until you discuss changing to another therapy.

Education is your biggest ally when it comes to the disease-modifying therapies. Knowing the potential side effects, setting realistic expectations, and troubleshooting potential problems will assist you in your goal to make DMTs a successful part of your management plan.

Neutralizing Antibodies (NAbs) and the Interferons

A small percentage of people can produce antibodies, which are a type of protein that may fight off the interferon that is trying to help them. In this scenario, the immune system seems to fend off the interferon with antibodies that may decrease the treatment's effectiveness. NAbs usually develop within twelve to eighteen months after the start of treatment. Researchers have discovered that not all the interferons generate the same amount of these antibodies. Also note that a percentage of those who develop NAbs continue to do well on a specific treatment. In others, NAbs may be present for only a short time period (such as a few months), and in these cases are probably insignificant.

Alert

If your treatment appears to be ineffective (even though you've been faithful to your injection schedule), your doctor may perform a test to see if NAbs are present in your bloodstream. Although individuals on interferon are not routinely tested for the presence of NAbs, researchers are currently trying to determine whether or not such routine testing might be advisable.

Paying for Treatment

The disease-modifying drugs for MS are very expensive, and thankfully, most insurance carriers in the United States provide some benefits for these treatments. How much coverage you get will depend on your particular policy, so before beginning any type of treatment it is important to ask the following questions:

- What type of insurance do I have?
- Is my treatment covered?
- What will my out-of-pocket costs be?

Not all insurance carriers cover prescription drugs, and those that do might have a list of specific drugs that they'll cover. You must also factor in your monthly copay amount, which will vary depending upon your plan.

Fact

In a 2007 survey of insured people with MS, more than two-thirds of the respondents expressed satisfaction with their insurance coverage, citing comprehensive coverage, overall affordability, and relatively low copays for expensive MS drug therapies as the major reasons for their satisfaction with the coverage.

Financial Assistance

Financial assistance is available from the drug manufacturers for those that qualify. You may also want to turn to Medicare or Medicaid or Social Security Disability Insurance. Following is a list of programs that may be of assistance.

Patient-Assistance Programs

In response to the growing cost of medicine, many pharmaceutical companies now sponsor patient assistance programs. These programs are helping patients who qualify receive medication free of charge. Qualifications vary from company to company, but most are based on income and lack of outpatient prescription coverage. Age is not a factor in order to qualify. To learn more, visit the various pharmaceutical companies online or call their toll-free number.

Pharmaceutical Assistance Programs

Many state governments play a substantial role in offering direct pharmaceutical assistance benefits to eligible residents. Most commonly, individual states offer substantial subsidies to low- and moderate-income seniors. About half these states include younger adults with disabilities among those who are eligible.

A majority of these programs are recognized within the federal Medicare Modernization Act (MMA) and are termed State Pharmaceutical Assistance Programs, or SPAPs.

In the past five years, a growing number of states have started offering state pharmaceutical discount programs. To see whether your state participates and, if so, what the specific eligibility requirements are, visit the National Conference of State Legislatures website (*www.ncsl.org*) or Medicare (*www.medicare.gov/spap.asp*).

Medicare Prescription Coverage

Medicare prescription drug coverage is insurance that covers both brand-name and generic prescription drugs at participating pharmacies in your area. Medicare prescription drug coverage provides protection for people who have very high drug costs or from unexpected prescription drug bills in the future.

Everyone with Medicare is eligible for this coverage, including those individuals under the age of sixty-five who get Medicare due to a disability. As with other insurance, if you join, generally you will pay a monthly premium, which varies by plan, and a yearly deductible ($0 to $265 in 2007). You will also pay a part of the cost of your prescriptions, including a copayment or coinsurance. Costs will vary depending on which drug plan you choose. Some plans may offer more coverage and additional drugs for a higher monthly premium. If you have limited income and resources, and you qualify for extra help, you may not have to pay a premium or deductible. You can apply or get more information by calling Social Security at 1-800-772-1213 (TTY 1-800-325-0778) or by visiting *www.ssa.gov* on the web.

Medicaid

Medicaid was designed to assist low-income families in providing health care for themselves and their children. It also covers certain individuals who fall below the federal poverty level. It covers hospital and doctor's visits, prenatal care, emergency room visits, drugs, and other treatments.

Other people who are eligible for Medicaid include low-income children under age six, low-income pregnant women, Supplemental Security Income recipients, adopted or foster children, specially protected groups, children under age nineteen whose family income is below federal poverty level, some Medicare beneficiaries, and other groups, as determined by each state. Most families that receive welfare probably have a social worker assigned to them, and this person will usually advise a family on its Medicaid eligibility. Your doctor will also be able to inform you about Medicaid. Depending on your state's rules, you may also be asked to pay a small part of the cost (copayment) for some medical services. For more information, visit *www.medicaid.gov* or call your local Social Security office for more information.

⎍ Essential

You may want to look to your community for assistance. There are community-based charitable organizations that may be able to assist you with your drug costs. The Benefits Check Up website at *www.benefitscheckup.org* is a great resource in helping you identify organizations and programs that can help.

If you're not insured, or your coverage is limited, putting your nose to the grindstone and investing some time in research can really pay off. There is an abundance of programs and organizations whose help you can enlist if you're having a hard time affording a treatment plan. The downside for a lot of people is investing hours filling out forms and plugging their way through the red tape, but your investment of time is an investment in your future.

People who are diagnosed with MS today are in a much better position than people who received the same diagnosis even twenty years ago. And while the new therapies require a commitment from you, they're your best line of defense right now. New and easier treatments are in the pipeline and are eagerly awaited by those in the MS community.

CHAPTER 7

The Relapse

PERHAPS THE MOST unwelcome event in relapsing-remitting multiple sclerosis is the relapse, which is usually the appearance of new symptoms or, less commonly, the worsening of old symptoms. Almost all people with multiple sclerosis experience relapses, except those with PPMS.

What Is a Relapse?

A relapse is a clinically significant event (meaning that it has outward signs and/or symptoms) caused by an MS lesion in your CNS. It is either the appearance of new symptoms or the worsening of symptoms that you already have. Relapses are also referred to as "exacerbations," "attacks," or "flares." Symptoms must last at least twenty-four hours and be separated from a previous relapse by at least one month to qualify as a true relapse.

Some relapses will be obvious to you. Losing feeling in your foot is an example of an obvious relapse. However, other relapses may not be as sudden or dramatic and you may just feel unusually tired. One way to truly identify a relapse is to have an MRI with gadolinium (a dye-like contrast material that is injected intravenously during the MRI). Gadolinium is drawn to areas of inflammation and "lights up" when a lesion is active. If you are having a definite relapse, inflammation is at work, and you are experiencing an attack, rather than feeling symptoms caused by older lesions.

 Fact

> In order for your neurologist to diagnose a relapse, your symptoms must show evidence of occurring in your CNS, and there must be no other possible cause of your symptoms, such as a fever or overheating. You and your doctor will also surmise whether or not your symptoms are disruptive to your daily life before he decides if treatment is necessary.

Is This the Real Thing?

If you think you're having a relapse, sit back and ask yourself a few questions. Am I overheated? Have I been exposed to anyone who has been ill lately? Have I been under a lot of stress? If the symptoms persist for more than a day, it's a good idea to call your doctor and let him know what's going on. The earlier you treat a relapse (should your doctor decide treatment is needed), the better chance you have of shortening its duration.

Symptoms that appear to be a relapse but don't meet the criteria for a true exacerbation are called pseudoexacerbations. They might feel like a relapse and look like a relapse, but they don't make the grade. There are many reasons symptoms can act up, but the most common reason is heat sensitivity.

Heat sensitivity occurs when the core body temperature of someone with MS increases—even just a half degree in body temperature can cause chronic symptoms to worsen. In the case of a pseudoexacerbation, when the body's temperature returns to normal, these symptoms disappear. Heat sensitivity can start when you're running a fever because of an infection (such as a cold, the flu, or a urinary tract infection), when you're outside on a hot day, or when you're being physically active in a warm environment.

Essential

The good news about pseudoexacerbations is that no damage is occurring to your CNS when you are experiencing symptoms. It is just a matter of cooling your body off and bringing down your core temperature until your symptoms subside. If your symptoms are caused by an infection, you may not feel better until the infection has resolved.

Stress and Other Causes for a Pseudoexacerbation

Even people without a chronic illness report feeling sapped when they're undergoing a great deal of stress. Many people with MS report intolerance for stress, and indeed, it may play a role in causing your symptoms to flare.

It's important to know when to take a timeout. Part of managing an illness is knowing when it's time to step back from the demands of everyday life and give yourself some time to rest and relax.

Alert

Relapses vary in their length and severity, but the first line of defense is to call your doctor and devise a plan to get the relapse under control. Knowing the difference between a true relapse and a pseudo-relapse will help you to decide when to make that call. Because medications are available that can help during a relapse, it is important to report new symptoms to your doctor right away.

Being extra tired can also cause your symptoms to flare, especially on those days when you've pushed yourself hard. Most people with MS know the feeling—it's something like hitting a wall, and like it or not, your body will demand that you give in to some rest and relaxation.

What Causes a Relapse?

Relapses are caused by the inflammation that occurs when your immune system attacks the myelin that surrounds nerves in your brain or spinal cord. When the myelin is attacked by immune cells, a lesion or an area of inflammation and eventual damage (demyelination) occurs, making the nerves less efficient in conducting signals. Your symptoms depend on the location of this lesion. For instance, inflammation in the cerebellum can cause loss of balance and coordination, while inflammation of the optic nerves can cause decreased vision.

Question

Can an infection cause a relapse?
No one knows, exactly, what happens before an attack, but attacks seem to occur more frequently after an infection, such as a viral infection of the upper respiratory tract. Several studies have shown that there is an increased risk of exacerbations in the first four weeks after an infection.

Some studies have sought to determine whether stress is a contributory factor in a relapse. The results of these studies are not definitive. There is also no clinical proof that trauma or surgery can trigger a relapse.

Another trigger for attacks occurs in women during the three months after the delivery of a child. It is important to recognize that the risk for an attack is *mildly* increased during this time and that pregnancy itself actually decreases the risk for attacks.

A relapse is typically unpredictable and occurs without warning. Until research fleshes out the cause of relapse in MS, the best advice is to learn to live with the uncertainty while maintaining an optimistic attitude. Of course, staying on track with your treatment plan can decrease the number of relapses you experience.

How Long Does a Relapse Last?

One of the most frustrating aspects of multiple sclerosis is its lack of predictability. Just as symptoms vary from person to person, the duration of an attack also varies, and not just from person to person, but also from one attack to another.

Generally, relapses tend to extinguish on their own within twelve weeks, but it can be much shorter than that, or even longer. Some relapses last just a few weeks while others may last up to six months. Some symptoms will go away completely while others may last indefinitely. In other words, once a relapse has resolved itself, some lingering symptoms may remain.

Relapses range from mild to severe. Some studies point to the fact that relapse frequency is highest in the first few years. This means that although you may have two attacks in a period of say, eighteen months, it does not necessarily foretell a dire outcome.

Treatment for Relapses

The treatment goal for a relapse is to stop the attack in its tracks and bring the individual with MS back to his pre-relapse condition. Most relapses actually resolve on their own, and often, especially in the early stages of the disease, the symptoms disappear once the inflammation has quieted down. It's possible you'll wake up one day and feel like your old self again, but you may also have some residual effects from the relapse, where a few of the symptoms hang on for a while, or perhaps even permanently.

Since most attacks resolve themselves, treating an attack with medication is not automatic. Your physician will try to determine how much the attack is interfering with your life or how severe the attack really is. It's important to keep track of any symptoms or attacks that occur. This record will help you to understand how your body is functioning, and it may also aid your doctor in following your disease course.

Your doctor may prescribe a round of corticosteroids, which have been the mainstay of treatment for the management of acute relapses for many years. Generally, corticosteroids are prescribed for relapses when the symptoms of the attack are impairing your day-to-day routine, such as problems with vision, strength, coordination, or walking.

Fact

Steroids are not generally used for maintenance therapy, although studies are under way to see if they may have some long-term benefit on disease progression. Some research suggests that this approach might reduce destruction in the CNS, although more evidence is needed before it can be recommended. Side effects can be adverse when used over a long period of time.

The Lowdown on Corticosteroids

When people hear the word corticosteroids, they often confuse the steroids used for treatment of MS with anabolic steroids, which athletes take to improve stamina and endurance. They are not the same type of drugs.

Corticosteroids are artificial hormones that simulate hormones produced in the human body by the adrenal glands. When used for exacerbations, steroids can reduce inflammation in the CNS, help suppress the immune system's attack on myelin by closing the blood-brain barrier, and even improve electrical conduction. Despite their effectiveness, they do not appear to improve the long-term course of the disease and can actually lose effectiveness if overused. The type of steroid you are prescribed will determine how it is administered. Steroids are either administered orally or through IV infusion. Some common corticosteroids are:

- **Deltasone (prednisone).** A corticosteroid that is generally given orally. Physicians usually slowly taper patients off prednisone and other steroids to avoid any withdrawal symptoms.
- **Solu-Medrol (methylprednisolone).** A corticosteroid that is administered by IV infusion. Solu-Medrol is used for multiple sclerosis in high intravenous doses. It is sometimes followed up with oral prednisone.
- **Decadron (dexamethasone).** A corticosteroid that is usually administered orally but may also be given by IV infusion.

IV infusions of steroids are sometimes given in a hospital on an inpatient basis for the duration of the treatment (three to five days) so that your reaction can be monitored. You can also go to a clinic or an infusion center, where you will be given the medicine while lying down in a bed or reclining in a chair. Arrangements can be made for a nurse to visit your home to administer the treatment, as well.

Alert

Sometimes your doctor may instruct you to taper down the dose of a corticosteroid before stopping it completely. Abruptly stopping steroids can cause symptoms such as weakness, dizziness, anxiety or loss of appetite in some people. Be sure to follow your doctor's orders and carefully follow the instructions on the label of your medication.

Steroid Tips

It's always nice to get tips from others who know what a particular treatment is like. Here are a few that may make your steroid treatments a bit more comfortable:

Before infusion starts:

- Drink a lot of water before your infusion. It makes your veins larger and easier to find when the IV line is inserted into your vein.
- Corticosteroids can cause stomach irritation if given on an empty stomach. Have a good meal before your treatment and take an over-the-counter stomach acid reducer during the course of your steroid treatment.
- Decide ahead of time which arm you prefer to be used for the IV. Depending on how long the treatment lasts, you may have the line in place for up to five days. You may prefer not to have your dominant hand be used for the line.

During infusion:

- Relax during the infusion treatments. Bring along a magazine or an iPod to pass the time.
- Sometimes the rate at which the medication is being administered may make your face flush or increase your heart rate. You can ask the nurse to slow down the rate of the infusion if you are feeling uncomfortable.

Following infusion:

- Food may taste strange for a few hours after your treatment. Some people even report a metallic taste in their mouth. Suck on some ice chips and stick to bland foods until the taste goes away.
- You might want to limit sweets for a few days as steroids may increase blood sugar levels. Steroids may cause water retention. To reduce bloating, avoid or limit salty foods during treatments.

- Solu-Medrol can make you feel anxious, agitated, and irritable, so you might want to stay home and relax rather than plan a day of activity. Steroids may also cause depression.
- If steroids cause insomnia, try different techniques to help you sleep or ask your doctor for medicine to help you.
- Steroids reduce your immune system's ability to fight infection, so avoid contact with people who have symptoms of colds or other viruses.

Realistic Expectations

For some folks, the corticosteroids work very well and within days they experience relief from their symptoms and have a renewed sense of energy. Quite a few people report that they feel focused and are suddenly ready to do battle with messy garages, thank you notes, and yard work. The goal in using steroids is to have people back on track as quickly as possible, and for many, steroids do the trick.

But drugs don't have the same level of effect for everyone. For some, the steroids fail to have the same benefit and instead, they must wait for the relapse to resolve itself while working with their doctor to manage difficult symptoms. If your relapse is severe and the steroids aren't working for you, your physician may discuss trying another treatment.

Essential

Until you've been prescribed steroids, it's hard to predict how your body will react. While some people may feel focused and energetic, others may feel wired and agitated. Steroids are known to cause extreme mood swings that can range from euphoria to depression. A good rule of thumb is to schedule some down time until you learn how you handle a medication.

Corticosteroid Side Effects

You've already learned about some of the side effects of steroids, such as mood swings and water retention. Following is a comprehensive list of side effects:

- Fluid retention
- Blurry vision
- Mood changes
- Insomnia
- Weight gain and redistribution of body fat
- A weakened immune system (temporarily)
- Acne (with prolonged use)
- Thinning of the skin (with prolonged use)
- Increased blood sugar (hyperglycemia)
- Thinning of bones and decreased blood flow to bones (especially with prolonged use)

You may want to troubleshoot potential side effects with your doctor and prepare ahead of time, but keep in mind that not everyone experiences side effects. Your experience may also differ each time you use steroids. Most people tolerate steroid treatment well in short intervals, although long-term use is not recommended because of potential serious side effects.

The Relapse Plan

Although relapses are an unwanted and uninvited guest, having a relapse plan will help you to prepare in advance for its potential arrival.

Talk to your doctor about her relapse protocol and make sure to ask her at what point you should call to let her know your symptoms have changed. Your plan should encompass a protocol for handling work and family responsibilities. Assume that you may need some time off, depending on how severe the relapse is. Decide now how you will handle talking to a boss, asking friends or family members for help, or changing your daily routine.

Have a relapse toolkit on hand full of things to relax and comfort you: good books, any over-the-counter medicines your doctor recommends, a gift certificate for a massage, takeout menus from your favorite restaurants, and a few DVDs you'd be happy to watch again. If rest is in order, your plan can incorporate some projects you've been meaning to get to such as sorting through and organizing photographs, cleaning out a filing cabinet, catching up on correspondence, or learning to play bridge. Turn the negative into a positive by putting the time to good use.

Your MS team is an ally when you're having a relapse. Call or get a referral to a physical therapist if you're experiencing muscle weakness, walking difficulty, or lack of coordination. For many people with an attack, the combined use of steroids and physical therapy may provide the quickest path for recovery. Get a referral to a psychologist or other mental health professional if you're experiencing depression or other psychological issues. Make a list of your symptoms—especially those that are most disruptive—and discuss them with your physician.

Fact

In 2006, Australian researchers studied the connection between MS relapses and stress, and found, not surprisingly, that people who were experiencing a relapse reported more stress. The study also showed that people who use social support (friends and family) to cope with stressors reduced their risk of relapse. However, there is no definitive proof that stress causes MS attacks.

Everyone deals with relapses in his own way. Because they're unpredictable, having a plan is a good idea. Because they're unwelcome, finding a coping strategy can help you over the hurdles. The use of disease-modifying therapies can cut relapse rates, but the reality is that you may face a setback from time to time. Until there is a cure, staying optimistic, adhering to a treatment plan, and planning for the unexpected is your best bet. Listening to and understanding your own unique body is also imperative. It's important to have a sense of control over the things you can control—such as the amount of sleep you're getting, your exercise regimen, the foods you eat—in short, your overall health and well-being.

Remission

Remission is defined as "the complete or partial recovery that follows an MS relapse." What this means is that the attack has resolved itself. It also means that some of the symptoms may stay with you on a permanent basis. More than likely, you will return to the baseline of functionality that existed before the attack, with or without new symptoms in tow. Some relapses leave damage in their wake in the form of plaques or scar tissue. Even with lingering symptoms, remissions bring some level of relief and a resumption of activities and routines for weeks, months, and even years.

Despite feeling "on track" again, for many, remissions come loaded with uncertainty. Some people report a certain amount of anxiety when they begin to take on more responsibility and independence after a difficult attack. Part of the anxiety stems from transitioning from the "ill" self to the "well" self. You may worry about how many former activities you can take on right now. You may worry about future attacks. For people with chronic illnesses there is never a shortage of things to worry about.

Recovery from a difficult attack isn't simple. You have to gently feel your way through each day, using good sense to determine what is realistic and what is not. It's still important to listen to your needs and incorporate flexibility into your schedule. There's also an adjustment to the "new normal," as life has undoubtedly gone on during your relapse and friends, family, and coworkers have been together, doing things, going places, and making decisions. You'll have to ease yourself back into their routines.

First and foremost, it is important *not* to try to make up for lost time of weeks and months of inactivity all at once. Pace yourself. Incorporate balance and good sense into your new routine.

Essential

Learning how to handle the emotional aspects of multiple sclerosis is just as important as dealing with the physical symptoms. *MS and Your Feelings* by Allison Shadday is a good resource for learning how to manage the emotional aspects of MS, including strategies for dealing with grieving, beating depression, and building self-esteem.

Ups and Downs of MS

Handling the ups and downs of MS can be challenging, and many find the emotional component of the disease to be just as troubling as the physical symptoms. And while life for all people has the tendency to be ever-changing, it is especially difficult for those with a chronic illness.

Each person handles the uncertainty of MS in her own way, but dealing successfully with the disease will mean developing and living by a strategy of self-care, tinged with optimism and a proactive approach. Seeking help from a professional—such as a psychotherapist or an occupational therapist—when you need it and staying on top of your treatment plan will go a long way in helping you to create a dependable emotional compass.

CHAPTER 8

Taking Charge

YOU HAVE EDUCATED yourself about the disease, are able to make informed decisions, and have specific goals in mind to manage your overall health. Once you understand the disease course—or how MS tends to behave for most people with the disease—you'll be able to create a management plan that allows you to put MS into proper perspective. In essence, it's a to-do list for well-being. It will emphasize getting the best health care you can, learning how to manage your days, and finding ways to cope with life's stresses.

Understanding the Disease Course

By now you've come to understand that in most cases, MS follows a pattern of periods of worsening followed by periods of remission and stability. The disease-modifying therapies are your best bet right now for prolonging remission and reducing relapses.

In general, the disease course in both relapsing-remitting multiple sclerosis (RRMS) and secondary progressive multiple sclerosis (SPMS) has the following characteristics:

- The disease begins as relapsing-remitting where patients experience exacerbations for several days to several weeks.
- Complete recovery from these attacks is typical at the onset of the disease.
- In some cases, as the disease progresses, the period between relapses increases and symptoms start to deteriorate slowly with or without relapses. This is called secondary progressive MS. However, some patients stay in a relapsing-remitting course for the rest of their lives, while others move into the secondary progressive form of the disease.
- About 10 percent of all multiple sclerosis–affected individuals experience chronic progression without relapses from onset of symptoms. This course is called primary progressive.
- Right now, the disease-modifying therapies are your best defense for relapsing forms of MS.

Researchers theorize that there are two components of MS—inflammation and degeneration. Inflammation is thought to cause relapses, while degeneration is believed to cause progression.

Early in the disease, there is probably a significant amount of inflammation that results in the relapsing-remitting course of the disease. Relapses, then, may be seen as a measure of how much inflammation is going on in the CNS.

Inflammation is thought to wane when the degenerative, or progressive, phase of the disease takes over and the relapsing -remitting pattern becomes less defined. People with MS may find that steroids or other treatments become less effective as the degenerative phase of the disease becomes more prominent. Researchers theorize that inflammation could be responsible for setting off this degenerative phase, and that's why targeting inflammation at the beginning of the disease is so important. Starting the DMTs early in the disease process has become an important cornerstone in MS treatment.

A Word about Primary Progressive MS (PPMS)

Primary progressive disease is characterized by a gradual progression of the disease from onset without relapses or remissions. There may be periods of a leveling off of disease activity and there may be good and bad days or weeks. PPMS differs from RRMS in other ways:

- Onset often begins later, in the late thirties or early forties.
- Initial disease activity may be in the spinal cord and not in the brain.
- PPMS may be less likely to show inflammation, which may explain why the disease-modifying therapies have not been shown to be particularly effective for PPMS.

It's important to note that having "progressive" MS does not necessarily mean severe disability or rapid worsening. Progression occurs, but in some people it may occur at a very slow pace over the course of years. While there are no FDA-approved disease-modifying treatments for PPMS, there are many useful strategies and treatments to help you manage.

Fact

When compared to relapsing-remitting MS or secondary progressive MS, people with primary progressive MS tend to have fewer and smaller lesions, fewer new lesions over time, and less enhancement with gadolinium, the marker that is injected before an MRI scan to show areas of inflammation.

Of course, it is impossible to predict what type of course the disease will take in any one person, but research has shown that this is a general pattern characteristic of the disease.

Creating a Strategic Plan

A management plan is a like a written instruction booklet that will assist you in seeing the big picture—treatment strategies, goals, and coping strategies are all part of the plan. Throughout this book, it's been suggested that you keep careful track of your medical records as well as using journals and calendars to record your feelings and thoughts, important appointments, and medication routines. In the same notebook, or perhaps a separate one, it is useful to outline your management plan so that you can turn to it when you need to identify a problem and decide best how to deal with it. Of course, your neurologist is the best person to guide you, but a management plan can help you stay on track. A good management plan will include the following components.

Goals

Make a list of goals you'd like to achieve, such as an exercise regimen or a nutritional plan. Also outline how you can best achieve these goals, such as joining a gym or enlisting the help of a nutritionist. Give yourself some time to implement a task but pinpoint a "do date."

Treatment

An outline of your treatment plan is helpful in managing your treatment goals. For example, if you're on one of the disease-modifying therapies, outline your injection schedule and list any questions or concerns you have for the neurologist. If injection-site problems are an issue, list it under side effects. For every concern you face, have a plan to address it and decide whom you should address it to.

Symptom Management

Keep a symptoms list with a strategy on how to manage each one. For example, if leg weakness has become an issue, you may want to talk to your neurologist about getting some physical therapy. Your goal here is to address and strategize each and every aspect of the disease that needs your attention.

Emotional Health

Keep track of your emotional health, too. Sometimes people get so bogged down in the myriad of details and appointments that they forget how important their psychological health is to their well-being. You may want to take note of your moods and identify stressors in your life. Have a strategy in mind to deal with your mental health issues, such as locating a therapist or someone who can help you alleviate stress.

A management plan is a good way to strategize the problems associated with a chronic illness. Your goal is to be organized and proactive when dealing with your health. If organization isn't your strength, get some help from a family member or a social worker.

Multidisciplinary Care

Chapter 5 discussed creating a management team. As part of your management plan, you'll have to identify which health professionals will best suit your strategy to address symptoms. Symptom management is essential to your care.

Rehabilitation Specialists

Whether you're looking to strengthen your muscles, improve your gait, or get help with occupational difficulties, these specialists have all kinds of strategies in tow to help you improve the quality of your life. From occupational and vocational specialists to physical therapists, they've got the tools to get you exercising or increase your performance at work. Take a look at your management plan to identify your symptoms or concerns and then page back to Chapter 5 to identify a specialist who can address the issue. Always discuss your ideas with your neurologist first.

Mental Health Professionals

Managing the emotional effects of chronic illness is just as important as taking care of the physical symptoms. It's also important to identify which symptoms are simply part of the ups and downs of

MS and which may be more pernicious. Depression, for example, is common in MS and might be more pervasive than simply having the blues.

A good therapist can guide you through the years, first helping you to tackle your diagnosis, for example, and then move on to other issues that may arise, such as job difficulties or family matters. A psychiatrist who is familiar with your psychological health is also imperative if depression is an issue for you. He may prescribe medications that can help you keep depression in check. Remember that depression isn't "failure to cope" but may be an indication something is amiss with the chemistry of your brain.

Social workers can help you identify your needs, such as transportation services, meals, and other community services, so be sure to keep them in mind as part of your overall management plan. A good plan is one in which you are vigilant in identifying your needs.

Primary Care Physicians

If you're not using your general medical doctor to manage your MS, be sure you see her on a regular basis for routine checkups and physicals. Don't forget that your general health is extremely important. Not everything that affects you physically is a result of MS; you'll still get colds and toothaches like everybody else.

In fact, as part of your management plan, you may want to turn over a new leaf when it comes to establishing good health habits. You want to be as strong and as healthy as possible, so if changing your diet or getting to the gym has been on your list, now would be a good time to make those changes. In addition to seeing your doctor regularly, schedule dentist appointments every six months. Consult a registered dietitian for tips on healthy eating. Other professionals, such as massage therapists, can also help you to maintain good health.

Creating a management plan is a way of charting your course. Learning to manage the disease is an ongoing process, but consistently taking stock of your condition and then identifying your needs will help you gain a measure of control and keep you on top of things from the get-go.

Essential

Getting involved in MS fundraising and government affairs is a great way to stay active and direct your energy toward an important cause. There are many legislative decisions that affect people with MS and other chronic illnesses, such as stem cell research and rights for the disabled. The NMSS has information on advocacy at *www.nationalmssociety.org/government-affairs-and-advocacy/index.aspx*.

Tips for Daily Living

Because MS varies s from person to person, no list of tips can include it all. The tips offered here, however, have been helpful to people with chronic illnesses over the years, not to mention people who don't have health issues to deal with. These tips focus on conserving energy.

Delegate Tasks

You've been meaning to do this anyway, right? Get the kids or other family members involved in chores. Make up a new list and hang it on the refrigerator door, breaking down chores and who's responsible for doing them.

Organize Tasks

Post-It notes are the miracle cure for busy people. Staying organized is your greatest time saver. Have shopping lists, chore lists, contact lists—and keep them all together in the same place. A large three-ring binder can be your best ally. They've got ruled paper for diaries, note keeping, and Post-It collections, pockets for notes and loose papers, and more than one section to keep different subjects separated. The best ones zip up and can be carried with you.

Let Go

As much as most people try, it's never been possible to do it all. Now is a good time to let go of any perfectionist attitudes and settle for less. What can you let go of? Does the house really need to be vacuumed three times a week? Can the car wait another week to be washed?

Clean the Clutter

Nothing takes up more time and energy than looking for things. The new buzz word for organization is "simplify." Buy large plastic containers at discount stores and use them to store things around the house that you're not using. Label them with their contents, such as "crafts," "financial paperwork," "Christmas decorations," and "photos." Then put them in an easy place to access, such as a storage closet or a basement. Purchase inexpensive shelving to get books off the floor, a filing cabinet for important documents, or a cabinet specifically designed for movies or CDs. Declutter and simplify! Clean out your drawers, give those old sweaters to a charitable organization, and throw those old coupons away. It's a good idea to tackle just one room at a time. Set a timer and commit to just fifteen minutes per day.

Fact

Not everyone is gifted with organizational skills, and if you fit that category, rally the troops! Perhaps you have a friend who can help you declutter. If not, hire a professional organizer. The number of these professionals has grown over the years. Depending on the size of the job, they can be in and out in a matter of days.

Part with the Old

Most people aren't particularly fond of change. Agree that you are eager to begin a new way of living—one that will simplify your life. As much as it hurts to part with your things, create piles of importance. One pile can be labeled "Haven't looked at in ten years," the next can be labeled "Still use occasionally." The trick is to be honest about how important something is. Be willing to part with those things that aren't used and are just taking up space.

Learn the Art of Zen

Zen cleaning involves agreeing to discard all the items in your life that have no use. While that might seem a little over the top to most people, it is a useful way to approach your decluttering task. It certainly eliminates those objects in your junk drawer that you cannot identify but are sure you might need one day. Zen cleaning ensures that everything in your life serves a function.

Create a Sacred Space

Everyone needs a place they go to for rest and relaxation, whether it's your bedroom, your garden, your workshop, or a corner of your kitchen. A sacred place is one where you can be yourself, and a place where MS is not allowed to venture. Have your earphones ready, your favorite music playing, or your tools handy. This is a place where you can catch your breath and be yourself for at least a few minutes every day.

Resetting Your Pace

You may still be going full throttle, but there may come a day where you have to adjust your pace—those days when fatigue is getting the best of you or a future event or appointment is on the horizon and you want to feel your best. Resetting your pace involves adopting flexibility into your life and adjusting your schedule to suit your needs. Following are some good ways to slow down.

Moderate Your Schedule

Try not to fit too much into one day. Working eight hours, going to the dry cleaners, and accepting an invitation to dinner with friends might work for some, but may not be realistic for others. Only you can decide what is reasonable, and it may take some time to figure out what your threshold is. If you agree to one very busy day, try to schedule less for the next day to give you some time to recover.

Get Rest

Researchers contend that people are simply not sleeping enough and its effects are pervasive. People with chronic illnesses need rest. Even if you're not in the dream state, you can find ways to relax and energize. Eight hours of sleep is still a good rule of thumb.

 Alert

> It's no secret that most people don't get enough sleep. People sleep an average of 6.9 hours per day, almost an hour less than a few decades ago. Since rest is an important way to combat fatigue in MS, you'll want to work with your physician to ensure that you're getting a good night's sleep. Those with sleep problems are more likely to feel stressed and tired.

Be Reasonable

It may be time to take an honest look at your life and decide what you can cut back on. Perhaps this assessment will help you to define what is putting you over the edge—too many volunteer committees, extra projects at work, or a carpooling commitment. Digging deep isn't easy; you might decide your job is too demanding or that you have to cut back on social engagements. The important thing is to be committed to a more reasonable pace and to prioritize your commitments.

Just Say No

Saying "no" is not an easy thing to do, but it's a strategy that all people have had to employ at one time or another. If you don't think you can help your mother move next Saturday, just say so. Offer to help her find someone else or try to find another way to assist her, such as packing her dishes or labeling boxes. Knowing your limits is healthy. This might be a good thing to discuss with a therapist, because although we'd all like to "just say no," actually doing it can prove to be difficult.

Fact

A recent study in the research journal *Sleep* examined the benefits of naps of various lengths and no naps at all. The results showed that a ten-minute nap produced the most benefit in terms of reduced sleepiness and improved cognitive performance. A nap lasting thirty minutes or longer is more likely to induce a period of grogginess when waking.

Pace Yourself

You may have a day where you're feeling especially energetic and so you try to take advantage of it by doing everything you've postponed for the past week or two. Overextending yourself one day may lead to overdoing, which you may pay for the next day. Pacing yourself is just as important on the good days as it is the bad.

Make your own list of tried-and-true tips on conserving your energy. And don't underestimate the power of the little things. Incorporating a timeout into your schedule every day is a little thing that can make a big difference. Letting someone else in your family take over the weekly dusting is another little thing that can make a big difference. Each thing you do to gain control over your life is another step toward self-empowerment.

Coping Strategies

It's one thing to get more sleep or delegate household chores; it's quite another to wrestle control of the emotional aspects of a chronic illness. Everyone employs certain coping mechanisms in life, but the important thing is to identify whether or not your strategies are healthy ones. A good rule of thumb is this: If it makes you feel better, it may be a good strategy. If it prolongs emotional discomfort or it allows you to avoid an issue, it may be time to find some new coping tools. Coping strategies refer to the specific efforts, both behavioral and psychological, that people use to tolerate or minimize stressful events. Two common coping strategies are behavioral strategies (used to alleviate stressful circumstances) and emotion-focused coping strategies (which involve efforts to regulate the emotional conse quences of stressful events). Research indicates that people use both types of strategies to combat more stressful events.

Behavioral strategies include things such as delegating tasks or starting an exercise routine, while psychological strategies include learning how to relax in stressful situations or training ourselves to respond differently to negative stimuli. You may deploy one or the other—sometimes both—depending on the situation.

Unhealthy Coping Mechanisms

Everyone adopts certain strategies to deal with difficult events. Here are a few to avoid:

- Lowering sights to what seems more achievable
- Mentally or physically avoiding something that causes distress
- Separating conflicting thoughts into mental compartments
- Refusing to acknowledge an event has occurred
- Avoiding emotion by focusing on facts and logic
- Subconsciously hiding uncomfortable thoughts
- Making a big problem small

Some of these unhealthy coping mechanisms actually serve you when you're trying to digest unsettling events, but in the long run, strategies such as avoidance or repression don't work. The person who uses stress as a reason to exercise (in a reasonable way) is learning and expressing a healthy coping mechanism. The person who turns to alcohol or food is using coping mechanisms that are both dangerous and unhealthy.

What are some good ways to cope with a chronic illness? Here are some healthy coping mechanisms, suggested by Dr. Andrew Kneier, who has worked with people with cancer for many years:

- **Face the reality of your illness.** Facing the issue is better for long-term coping, although a healthy dose of denial is common at diagnosis.
- **Maintain hope and optimism.**
- **Express your emotions.** Express both negative and positive emotions.
- **Reach out for support.** Studies show that people who find social support networks, such as support groups, fare better than those who do not.
- **Adopt a participatory stance.** This means empowering oneself by participating in treatment and decision-making.
- **Find a positive meaning in your illness.** Not always an easy thing to do, but helping others to cope and overcome adversity is one way to bring meaning to your circumstances.
- **Connect spiritually.** No matter what your beliefs are, connecting to something greater than yourself (even if it's hope, nature, or friendship) may be beneficial to your health.
- **Maintain self-esteem.** Finding ways to improve your self-confidence and maintaining a strong and positive sense of self is crucial. Hobbies, developing new skills and maintaining healthy relationships are just a few of the ways you can build self-esteem.

These coping strategies may not be right for everyone. It's best to see a therapist and decide what works best for you. It's important to work through the emotional aspects while keeping perspective. The often-heard statement "You are not your illness" is tried and true.

Balancing your illness with the other aspects of your life is key to a healthy emotional disposition.

Essential

Art therapy has been found to offer many benefits in auto-immune and other chronic disorders and has been used as therapy for people with neurological conditions. This type of therapy involves expressing yourself through artistic and creative means. Experts say it can improve the physical, mental, and emotional well-being of patients. For more information, visit *www.arttherapy.org*.

Planning Ahead

With one foot firmly planted in the present, you must also look ahead to your future when it comes to financial planning, social support, and career plans. That's something everyone should do, and people living with chronic illnesses have a particular need to lay the groundwork for the future. Those who are newly diagnosed or are experiencing changes in their MS should seek to reduce their anxiety about what lies ahead by addressing potential and practical issues.

Financial Planning

If you don't have one already, now may be a great time to find a competent financial advisor who will take a look at your financial profile and will help you maximize your worth through sound investing or saving. They also help their clients prepare and invest for long-term goals such as retirement. A well-chosen advisor can be an important ally in creating and carrying out a long-term financial plan. Referrals from friends and family are a good place to start, but it's important to do your homework. Pick up a good book that can instruct you on selecting the right financial advisor.

It's also important to become familiar with your state's social security and disability programs. While you might not ever need these services, you should understand how the programs work.

Alert

Financial experts say that 55 percent of American adults don't have a will. When people die without wills, it's up to the state to decide how their assets will be distributed, which may not reflect their desires. It's important for everyone to consider estate planning when looking toward the future.

Career Planning

People with MS should be open to re-evaluating their roles in the workplace as often as needed. While almost half of the people with MS retain employment after living with the disease for twelve years, flexibility, creativity, and adaptation are important factors in their success. New laws and changing attitudes have also made it easier for people with chronic illnesses to build or maintain their careers. Equally important is your ability to change the type of work you do if the need arises. A personal trainer who has issues with muscle weakness, for example, may want to see a vocational rehabilitation specialist to explore other career avenues.

Support Network

Planning ahead also includes building a network to support you if the going gets tough, whether it's a neighbor who's willing to shovel your driveway, a coworker who can cover for you in a pinch, or a local transportation service to get you to an appointment. Planning ahead means being resourceful and knowing what's available in your area. A community social worker can be helpful in outlining available services.

You hear so much about optimism when it comes to chronic illness, and indeed maintaining hope and a positive outlook are beneficial aspects to your well-being. But optimism must be tinged with practicality. Planning ahead might mean sticking your big toe into the pool of "what if" but it's a necessary dip into uncertainty. Being prepared for whatever the future brings serves to quell your fears. Taking charge and taking care of tomorrow can bring that much needed peace of mind today.

CHAPTER 9

Managing Symptoms

THE LIST OF symptoms for MS can look a little daunting at first glance, but remember that most people only experience a few. Since symptoms are unpredictable and vary from person to person, you may only choose to read about those symptoms that apply specifically to you. Symptoms also vary in intensity; some symptoms are not particularly troublesome and may not call for treatment. The good news is that symptom management in MS has come a long way. As research has begun to uncover the mysteries of the disease, symptoms are better understood and treated.

Fatigue

Fatigue in MS is extremely common, affecting up to 90 percent of people with the disease, and is described as the worst symptom by almost one-third of people with MS. MS fatigue is not normal fatigue; experts describe it as "deadening." One person described it as running a marathon in a suit of armor. It can vary from day to day, but it is particularly frustrating when you lack the physical or mental energy to get things done, so it's imperative to address it with your doctor.

The cause of fatigue in MS is not yet fully understood. It differs from ordinary fatigue in the following ways:

- It comes on much faster than ordinary fatigue upon exertion, even doing simple activities such as writing or walking.
- There is little correlation to the amount of energy expended and the degree of fatigue.
- MS fatigue takes longer to resolve than ordinary fatigue.
- MS fatigue can cause neurological symptoms to appear.

MS fatigue can be thought of in two ways: primary fatigue and secondary fatigue. Primary fatigue appears to be caused by the disease process itself and is a result of the demyelination in the CNS. Terms such as *lassitude fatigue* (fatigue experienced during activity), *heat intolerance* (symptoms brought on by hot weather or raising of the body temperature), and *localized fatigue* (nerves of individual muscle groups that tire with use) figure in to primary fatigue.

Secondary fatigue refers to the tiredness or weakness that occurs that is not directly related to the disease process, but instead occurs as a result of your symptoms. Sleep disturbances, medications, depression, lack of physical activity, and poor nutrition also come into play.

Essential

Your goal should be to identify troublesome symptoms and be proactive about them. If fatigue is making a trip to the mall seem like an insurmountable task, then it needs to be addressed. The overall goal of symptom management is to increase your quality of life.

Fatigue is one of the most underreported symptoms in MS because many people unknowingly accept it as an inevitable and untreatable consequence of having MS. It is important to tell your doctor that you are experiencing fatigue, even when other symptoms seem more obvious.

Getting a Handle on Primary Fatigue

Researchers believe that primary fatigue is caused by poor nerve conduction resulting from the demyelination process. It is not a result of anything you're doing, but occurs because your body is working a whole lot harder to transmit messages between your brain and other parts of your body.

While there are no specific treatments for primary fatigue, there are some medications that may provide some relief. If one medication doesn't seem to work for you, talk to your doctor about trying another. Here are some commonly used medications prescribed for fatigue:

- **Provigil (modafinil).** This drug is usually used to treat narcolepsy (a sleep disorder) but some drug trials found that it also reduced the fatigue associated with MS in some people.
- **Amantadine.** This is an antiviral medication that is also prescribed for fatigue in MS.
- **Ritalin.** This stimulant is often prescribed for people with ADHD, but may also be helpful for people coping with MS fatigue.
- **Prozac (fluoxetine).** This antidepressant has also been found to alleviate fatigue in some people with MS.

Once people learn to identify MS fatigue and realize there are ways to combat it, they are eager to move past this sometimes disabling symptom. Talk to your physician about some of the treatments used for fatigue. It may take some trial and error until you find a medication that works best for you.

Getting a Handle on Secondary Fatigue

Secondary fatigue is primarily caused by your symptoms. If you have muscle weakness in your legs, for example, walking down a long corridor at the airport may tire you out before you even get on the airplane. You'll have to problem-solve to conserve energy, which may mean requesting a wheelchair to get from the check-in counter to the gate. While this may be an uncomfortable solution at first, think of it as an investment in your future and your quality of life. Why feel fatigued when you get to your destination if you could have conserved that energy in the first place? Problem solving takes creativity, but it also takes flexibility.

You may also have to tackle problems with self-image, too, and rethink your ideas about assistive technology (AT), such as wheelchairs, scooters, and canes. These devices exist to make life easier for those who need assistance, and they work wonders for those who are trying to conserve their energy. Don't entertain the idea that you're "giving in." In reality, you're making a wise choice: you're saving your energy so that you're ready to enjoy and tackle the important things in your life.

℞ Question

Where can I learn more about assistive technology?
Assistive technology (AT) can open doors and break down barriers for people with disabilities and chronic illnesses. To familiarize yourself with the various gadgets available, visit these websites: *www.abledata.com* and *www .independentliving.com*. Their products include everything from canes to jar openers to jewelry.

Managing your time and energy is essential to getting a handle on fatigue. Developing strategies to offset the effects of fatigue will enable you to participate fully in life. Here's a list of tips to get you started:

- **Prioritize.** Of all the things that compete for your time and attention, choose those that you value most. Agree to expend a lot of your time and energy on those things that top your list, while giving other things less of your time. MS may force you to redefine what is important to you, including yourself.

- **Strategize.** Once you've got a handle on your priorities, you must come up with effective ways to handle the physical and mental tasks associated with them. Creativity is the key here. Once you figure out what you want done, you can strategize on how it gets done. Most of all, be willing to change your strategy if one isn't working for you.
- **Collaborate.** This means brainstorming with others to find ways to make your environment more accessible and organized. Ask your employer to move your office to a more convenient location. Ask family members to help you get your workshop organized. There are thousands of ways to save time and energy; you may be surprised by what sort of ideas you can come up with.

Essential

If you'd like to add some energy-saving ideas to your cache, check out the book *300 Tips for Making Life with Multiple Sclerosis Easier,* 2nd edition. Author Shelley Peterman peddles some great ideas here, such as meal preparation, ways to improve memory and concentration, grooming tips, and travel ideas.

Other Energy Sappers

There are other causes of MS fatigue, including sleep disturbances, medications, depression, lack of physical activity, and poor nutrition. Figuring out which of these areas you need to focus on can be a little challenging, but tackling each potential cause one at a time can help you figure out which ones are robbing you of energy.

Some of the medications prescribed for MS can cause insomnia, so be sure to go over your meds with your doctor and discuss which ones may be causing the problem. The interferons (Avonex, Betaseron, and Rebif) are known to cause fatigue, especially at the beginning of treatment. Other medications that cause drowsiness include Neurontin (gabapentin, for pain), Valium (diazepam, for spasticity), and antidepressants (for depression). Many other drugs in your MS arsenal can cause drowsiness, so check with your doctor if fatigue continues to be a problem for you. She may suggest changing your medication schedule or switching you to another type of drug.

Alert

Studies show that people with insomnia are four times more likely to suffer from depression than those without insomnia. Insomnia is also associated with anxiety and drug and alcohol abuse, along with injury and accidents. It's important to make the correlation between sleep and health and seek help if insomnia lasts longer than a week.

The inability to fall asleep or to stay asleep, called insomnia, is the most common sleep disorder. Many people with multiple sclerosis complain of insomnia or broken sleep patterns. Let's look at the most common causes:

- **Symptoms.** Symptoms such as muscle stiffness, muscle spasms, and frequent urination can interrupt your sleep.
- **Stress and depression.** Tossing and turning all night might be an indication that you're not getting a handle on stress. Depression can also keep people from falling asleep, especially if they have irregular sleep habits, such as sleeping too much during the daytime.
- **Drugs.** Corticosteroids (used to treat relapses) are known to give people an energy boost and sometimes keep them from sleeping, too.

- **Lack of exercise.** Known as deconditioning, a lack of exercise may worsen MS fatigue. Likewise, a regular exercise program may be an excellent, "nondrug" approach to treating MS fatigue.
- **Nutrition.** Poor nutrition can sap you of much-needed energy. Getting the right vitamins and minerals into your body will help you function at your optimal level.

Learning to rethink your activities and routines to cope with MS fatigue is often done by trial and error. The truth is, most people who have fatigue issues figure out for themselves what works best for them—and sometimes they learn the hard way. A good rule of thumb is to pay attention to what your body is telling you. Sometimes a few minutes rest will buy you some energy; other times, calling it a day might be in order.

Spasticity

Spasticity results from increased muscle tone as a result of demyelination in the CNS. It is a state whereby the muscles remain contracted and resist passive movement when induced by an external force—such as your doctor pushing against your hands. Spasticity is most common in the legs and may be associated with underlying weakness in the muscles, which can cause problems with walking. Spasticity is treated with medication, stretching, and education. Your doctor may also check to see if there is an underlying condition that may be triggering it, such as a urinary tract infection or bowel distention.

There are several drugs in your doctor's arsenal that can help, including Lioresal (baclofen) and Zanaflex (tizanidine). Other drugs that may be helpful include Neurontin (gabapentin) and Klonopin (clonazepam). Stretching exercises and learning the correct positions for lying and sitting can have value as well. A physical therapist is an important resource for nonmedication therapies for spasticity. More aggressive therapies for spasticity include injections of Botox (botulinum toxin) into stiff muscles or insertion of tubing into the spinal canal to deliver baclofen directly to the nerves (intrathecal baclofen pump).

Ataxia and Tremor

Ataxia is a lack of (or reduction in) coordination and may be associated with tremor, which means involuntary movement of a body part, such as an arm. Both can affect walking and limb function, as well as the ability to balance while standing or sitting. As in spasticity, drug treatment and patient education are important factors in treating these symptoms, but options to this date are limited to minimizing the effects of ataxia and tremor rather than eliminating them. There are several drugs used in treating these symptoms, including Atarax (hydroxyzine) (an antihistamine), Klonopin (clonazepam), and Topamax (topiramate). Most of the medications for tremor and ataxia cause drowsiness.

Fact

Lifestyle changes may help to manage some of the symptoms of tremor. Since caffeine can amplify tremor, avoiding or limiting coffee, tea, and chocolate intake is a good idea. Ask your doctor about some over-the-counter medications that may aggravate symptoms, such as certain cough syrups and allergy medications. Yoga, meditation, and other relaxation techniques can help relieve stress, which makes tremors worse.

An occupational therapist can help you improve your posture and maximize stability during activities. Studies show that attaching weights to your wrists or ankles (to assist with stability during activity) also has some benefit.

Bladder Dysfunction

Since bladder function is connected to three different levels of the CNS, it's not surprising that bladder problems are fairly common in MS. Urinary urgency and frequency are the most common symptoms. Other symptoms include difficulty initiating or completing urination and urinary incontinence. The management of bladder dysfunction involves two components: drug treatment and/or catheterization. If you're experiencing bladder problems you're not alone: up to 90 percent of people with MS have this symptom at one time or another. There are quite a few coping strategies you can add to your MS toolbox to help manage this symptom—which for many, can be taxing both psychologically and physically.

Drug treatments target the mechanisms in your bladder that cause the dysfunction—a series of interconnected nerves and muscles that coordinate the muscle contraction and relaxation necessary for normal bladder control. Different drugs target different symptoms.

Most often, problems emptying the bladder completely cause you to feel urinary frequency or urgency. You may even run to the bathroom and find that nothing happens when you get there. Lioresal (baclofen) may be able to help, as well as intermittent self-catheterization (ISC), which might sound a little scary at first, but most people come to appreciate the comfort and security it provides. For many, it's also easy to do (believe it or not). It involves inserting a catheter into the bladder and emptying the urine into the toilet. In some cases, ISC becomes a form of physical therapy and actually resolves the problem within a matter of weeks or months.

Urinary tract infections (UTIs) are often the unfavorable consequence of a bladder that doesn't fully empty, so it's important to get a handle on bladder problems. UTIs are very common in MS, so your doctor will probably check for them (with a quick urine test) if your symptoms flare up. An unchecked UTI can pose a serious risk to your health. The signs aren't always obvious, but some of the symptoms of a UTI are painful urination, frequent urination, and foul-smelling urine. UTIs are treated with a course of antibiotics.

A storage problem occurs when the bladder is unable to retain urine when it accumulates. Instead of expanding when urine collects, the bladder contracts, which can make you feel as if you have an urgent need to go to the bathroom all of the time. It can also interfere with a good night's sleep. Fortunately, there are several medications you can try that can calm your bladder down, including Ditropan (oxybutynin), Vesicare (solifenacin succinate), Detrol (tolterodine), and others. See your urologist or neurologist for help with these problems.

Essential

Don't cut down on your fluid intake as a way of managing bladder problems. When you don't drink enough, urine becomes very concentrated, does not flow as readily, and can lead to infection. It may make sense for you to drink the standard eight glasses a day if you're experiencing bladder problems. Good bladder management contributes to your quality of life and also prevents more serious complications from developing.

Bowel Problems

Constipation is common in MS and can occur as a result of a loss of sensation that signals you when it's time to use the bathroom. Similarly, the loss of sensation may result in an overactive bowel, and sometimes (though rare) a lack of bowel control. Problems with the bowel can occur with bladder dysfunction or by themselves.

It's important to find the root cause of any bowel problems. Sometimes, making a simple lifestyle change—drinking more water, increasing fiber intake, or taking a stool softener—can help ease some of the problems such as constipation and hard stools. A well-balanced diet and a regular exercise regimen are also treatment strategies. Be sure to talk to your doctor about any bowel problems you are experiencing. If he rules out other causes, there are some medications available to help with the symptoms caused by MS.

Visual Changes

For many people, a problem with vision is the first MS symptom. Vision problems are not uncommon, affecting up to 80 percent of people with the disease. The symptoms affect either your vision or the movement of the eye itself. Keep in mind that while vision problems are common in MS, they rarely result in permanent vision loss.

 Fact

> Optic neuritis typically affects people aged between fifteen and fifty years of age. In this age group, studies indicate that more than 50 percent of patients will be diagnosed with multiple sclerosis within fifteen years after a first bout with optic neuritis. As with MS, women are about twice as likely as men to present with ON and the prevalence in Caucasian people is higher than in other racial groups.

Optic Neuritis (ON)

Optic neuritis (inflammation of the optic nerve caused by demyelination) is the most common visual disorder and can cause an array of symptoms including vision loss in one eye, pain behind an eye, blind spots in the visual field, faded or washed-out color vision, and other problems. The visual deficit may worsen over a period of approximately seven days, and then typically remains stable for three to eight weeks, followed by gradual visual improvement. The great majority of patients with optic neuritis will recover much of their vision within six months of the onset of ON. Your neurologist may prescribe intravenous corticosteroids, as they've been shown to significantly increase the rate of the recovery from ON. If visual loss is relatively mild and manageable, the best alternative is probably to wait for the episode to remit on its own. It is not uncommon for a person to experience recurring episodes of ON and some residual effects may remain after the episode has cleared up, such as changes in color vision.

Alert

The symptoms of ON can flare up if your body is overheated from exercise, hot weather, or fever (an occurrence called Uhthoff's phenomenon). This is an example of a pseudorelapse and the symptoms usually clear up once your body temperature goes back to normal. Fatigue may also provoke symptoms from a previous episode of ON.

Eye Movement Problems

These problems refer to the movement of the eye and prove to be a complicated area of neurology. As with other MS problems, the difficulties can be subtle or marked. People with MS can experience problems when moving their eyes rapidly from side to side, for example, or when trying to follow the path of a moving object. Others experience involuntary eye movement. The more common eye movement problems in MS are diplopia and nystagmus.

Diplopia

Diplopia occurs when complex eye movements are out of sync. In other words, each eye has a mind of its own and the result is double vision. It's caused by decreased nerve input to the eye muscles. When the images are not properly fused, the person perceives a double image. Double vision may increase with fatigue or overuse of the eyes (such as extended reading) and improve with rest. Resting the eyes periodically throughout the day can be beneficial.

Diplopia usually resolves without treatment. In some cases, it is treated with a short course of corticosteroids. Temporarily patching one eye while trying to drive or read will also stop the double image.

Surgery or special prescription glasses in more severe cases are also options that should be discussed with your eye specialist.

Nystagmus

Another relatively common visual finding in MS is nystagmus, uncontrolled horizontal or vertical eye movements in one or both eyes. Nystagmus may be mild, only occurring when the person looks to the side, or it may be severe enough to impair vision. It does not always cause noticeable symptoms, and is a painless problem. Some drugs and special prisms have been reported to be successful in treating the visual deficits caused by nystagmus and another related eye movement disorder called opsoclonus, which causes "jumping vision." Corticosteroids may also be helpful in treating nystagmus, or the problem may resolve on its own. Baclofen, Klonopin, and Neurontin may alleviate nystagmus in some people.

Essential

Low-vision specialists and behavioral optometrists are licensed doctors of optometry who are trained in the examination and management of patients with visual impairments. Their services do not offer a cure for the causes of low vision, but they do help the patient learn how to utilize his remaining vision to its fullest potential. Check out www .lowvision.org for more information.

Other problems that can occur as a result of visual disturbances are dizziness, nausea, loss of balance, and disorientation, so getting a handle on eye problems is essential. Doctors who treat eye disturbances are low-vision specialists, ophthalmologists, and optometrists.

Swallowing and Speech Dysfunction

Swallowing problems are not uncommon in MS, and they are often associated with speech problems. If you're experiencing swallowing or speech problems, it's because you have an area of damaged nerves that normally aid in performing these tasks. Lesions in the brain can cause several different types of changes in normal speech patterns. Some of the symptoms are as follows:

- Unexplained recurrent lung infections
- The feeling that food is being lodged in your throat
- Coughing or choking when eating
- Unexplained malnutrition or dehydration
- Weight loss

Your doctor will try to identify the location of your problem by doing a physical exam during which he'll pay particular attention to how your tongue and neck muscles are functioning. He may also order a test called a modified barium swallow where you drink or eat various consistencies of contrast and have a special imaging machine take pictures to trace the path of the contrast material. It is important to determine whether the swallowing problems are due to MS or other medical conditions.

Swallowing Problems

Swallowing difficulties can cause secondary problems including pneumonia and malnutrition. This happens when food or liquids are inhaled into the trachea instead of going down to the esophagus and into the stomach. In the lungs, the inhaled food or liquids can cause pneumonia or abscesses. Because an adequate amount of food is not reaching the stomach, dehydration or malnutrition can also occur.

A speech therapist usually treats swallowing problems. Changes in diet, positioning of the head when eating or drinking, and exercises may be recommended to improve swallowing. In the most severe cases, a feeding tube may be inserted right into the stomach to provide nutrients.

Here are a few of the tips that can help improve swallowing function:

- Try to swallow frequently, alternating between food and liquid. Swallow two to three times per bite.
- Drink plenty of fluids.
- Eat soft foods such as applesauce, mashed potatoes, Jell-O, and pudding. Puree foods in a blender.
- Crush pills and sprinkle them on a tablespoon of applesauce instead of swallowing them with water. Some pills should not be crushed, so be sure to check with your pharmacist first.
- Eat slowly. Make sure to cut your food up into small pieces.

Finding a good speech/language therapist is important when you're trying to handle swallowing problems. They can teach you swallowing exercises that improve muscle coordination during swallowing. They can also recommend modifications in the way you eat or the consistency of the foods you eat.

Speech Problems

Two common speech problems in MS are scanning and the slurring of words. Scanning produces speech in which the rhythm or cadence is disrupted with long pauses in between words or syllables. Slurring of words occurs because muscles in the tongue, lip, and mouth become weak. Some of the symptoms of speech problems include the following:

- Imprecise or slower speech
- Speaking in a low volume
- Difficulty with resonance and pitch control
- Long pauses between words or syllables of words
- Difficulty in understanding what is being said and an inability to recall grammar or vocabulary

A speech/language therapist or pathologist can help people with MS to improve speech patterns and enunciation. For those with severe speech problems, communication aids such as alphabet cards or hand-held communicators are useful.

Speech problems can run the gamut from very mild to severe. Troublesome speech problems can make it difficult to form words properly. It's important to note that, like any symptom in MS, speech problems can come and go, sometimes in the space of a few hours.

Sexual Problems

Intimacy with your partner is part of a fulfilling life. Sometimes, though, the physical changes people experience and the psychological impact of these symptoms can make it difficult for people with MS to feel enthusiastic about their sex lives. The good news is that there are quite a few strategies that can help you manage these difficulties and get your relationship back on track.

Some of the most common changes in sexual function are a direct result of neurologic changes (such as spasticity or bladder problems), or they can be a result of psychological problems, such as not feeling very sexy during a relapse. Medications can also cause changes in libido.

Sexual problems in MS are defined as primary, secondary, and tertiary. Primary problems are the direct result of the disease affecting the nerves in your CNS and can result in a decrease in sex drive, difficulty reaching an orgasm or maintaining an erection, or numbness, pain, or increased sensitivity in the vaginal area. A decrease in vaginal lubrication can also occur.

Because sexual arousal begins in the CNS, changes to the nerve pathways can directly impair sexual functioning. But the secondary problems or psychological effects can be just as devastating. Fatigue can put a damper on your sex life and sensory problems can make you oversensitive to contact. Bowel and bladder problems can create a roadblock to intimacy, as can difficulty with movements or positions involved in sex because of pain or muscle spasms.

Tertiary problems are caused by the psychological problems rooted in self-image. Depression, changes in self-image, and lack of confidence can dampen your moods and sex drive.

There are all kinds of ways (whether directly or indirectly) for sexual dysfunction to sneak into your relationship, so it's important to speak to your doctor if you have questions or concerns. Medication may be useful in tackling some of the problems. Communication with your partner is also imperative. Enlisting the help of a therapist is also important; she may be able to shed some light on the psychological barriers that may be preventing you from having intimate relations with your partner.

Medications and Treatments for Men

Men report failure to have an erection as their primary problem. Here are some treatments to consider:

- **Oral medications.** Viagra (sildenafil) and other medications can help men achieve and maintain erections, and are effective for about 50 percent of men with MS.
- **Injectable medications.** These medications are injected into the base of the penis. Unlike oral medications, the injectable medications produce an erection within a couple of minutes.
- **Penile treatments.** A doctor can insert various devices into the penis to assist with erections.
- **Muscle relaxants and pain medication.** These medications can be used to help spasms and pain that may interfere with sex.

Some treatments, such as penile implants, are more invasive than others, but your physician can assist you in finding an option that you're comfortable with.

Medications and Treatments for Women

Women with MS report failure to achieve an orgasm and lack of sex drive as among their most troublesome sexual symptoms. Here are some treatments to consider:

- **Vaginal lubricants.** These over-the-counter gels can help with vaginal dryness. It's important to use an adequate amount.

- **Timing.** If fatigue is an issue, try having sex at different times during the day.
- **Vibrators.** These electronic devices can help if impaired sensation or slow arousal is an issue.
- **Muscle relaxants and pain medication.** If muscle spasms or pain are getting in the way, these medications can be very helpful.
- **Positioning.** Try different sexual positions to find one that works best for you and your partner. This is often helpful for people who have a decrease in the range of motion in their arms and legs from spasticity or muscle weakness.
- **Bladder control.** If bladder control is an issue for either sex, self-catheterization, going to the bathroom before sex, or medication can be used to help control the symptoms.

Alert

Don't forget that medication can decrease libido. Some of the drugs used for depression and bladder control can cause some sexual problems. Go over your list of medications with your doctor. Sometimes drugs can be substituted with others that have fewer sexual side effects.

Recent studies have shown that a woman's concept of sexuality and her sexual identity are more complex than those of men. Therefore, interventions for women are more relationship focused and counseling is often recommended.

Communication Is Key

Being able to talk about sex is often the biggest obstacle to tackling sexual dysfunction. Learning to communicate (no matter how uncomfortable at first) with your partner and your health care team can empower you to approach these problems with a sense of knowledge and creativity.

Picking an appropriate time to approach your partner is imperative. The best time to approach someone for a talk about your sex life isn't when either one of you is busy or tired. Pick a time when you're both relaxed and enjoying a moment together.

Question

Does health insurance cover sex therapy?
Some policies do. If you select a therapist, call her to check. If payment cannot be worked out through insurance, many therapists can adjust their fees. Sex therapy clinics tend to be less expensive than private therapists. Call your local hospital or university medical center to see if they have a sex therapy clinic.

Being a good listener is also a good rule of thumb, albeit a difficult task for some people. Agree not to interrupt or talk over your partner. Remember to be specific when you articulate your concerns. If there's something new you'd like to try—a new position or medication—state it clearly and confidently. Telling your partner what feels good or what doesn't feel good during intimacy is also essential for an intimate relationship.

Although it can be uncomfortable at first, good communication with your health care team about sexual dysfunction is essential. You don't have to suffer in silence when there is a plethora of strategies that can help you. Since sexual dysfunction is common in MS, your doctor has had this conversation many times before.

Sensory Symptoms and Pain

Sensory symptoms can be annoying (and they're also very common) but the good news is that they're often not serious. They may not be indicative of disease progression, and, generally, they are not incapacitating. There is a wide range of sensory symptoms including a pins-and-needles feeling in the arms or legs (and other places), burning or itching skin, changes in how you interpret hot and cold, and others. Unless these symptoms are significantly interfering with your life, your doctor will probably elect not to treat them, although a short course of corticosteroids can be used in cases where the symptoms recently began and are particularly troublesome.

Pain and MS

Twenty years ago doctors believed that pain was not an issue in MS. These days, there is no question that people with MS can experience pain. Recent studies show that neuropathic pain (pain caused by problems in the nervous system) occurs in about 50 percent of people with MS sometime during the course of the disease.

Of course, no two people experience pain in the same way. For some, pain may be fleeting and short-lived, whereas for others, it can be a daily nuisance. Even mild changes in sensations can have an impact on daily life, so it is important that pain is acknowledged and managed. Pain, by the way, is defined as anything that causes you mental or physical discomfort. For some, pain can be exhausting, but it also causes fear, distress, and frustration. This is one of the symptoms you'll want to get a handle on right away.

Pain in MS falls into two categories: primary pain and secondary pain. Primary pain is caused by nerve damage, whereas secondary pain is indirectly caused by MS symptoms.

Primary Pain

Primary pain is also called neuropathic pain and is caused by damage to the nerves. There are several types of primary pain:

- Trigeminal neuralgia is an intense, sharp, stabbing facial pain and is usually short-lived. It is relatively rare in MS.
- Lhermitte's sign is a sudden sensation like an electric shock that spreads to the arms or legs and is triggered when the neck is bent forward.

- Dysesthesias are the most common type of pain and include burning sensations in your arms, legs, or trunk, or the "MS hug"—a "girdling," bandlike feeling around your chest or midsection.

It is important that any pain you are experiencing is correctly diagnosed and properly treated. There are more available drugs and other therapies today for MS pain than ever before and new treatments are in the pipeline.

Essential

Only a small number of people with MS will develop trigeminal neuralgia (4 percent). The condition can be very painful and tends to recur. The pain is usually relieved by anticonvulsant or antiseizure medicine, and for those cases that don't seem to be responding to medication, surgery is an option.

Treatment

Your neurologist may try to treat your neuropathic pain with medication, but you may have to try several drugs to see which one works best for you. The trick is to find relief with the fewest number of medication side effects. There are currently no medications specifically approved for MS pain, but the following drugs have been used with some success:

- Cymbalta (duloxetine hydrochloride) was approved by the FDA for the treatment of depression and the treatment of pain associated with diabetic peripheral neuropathy. Although not specifically approved for use in MS, it may be effective for MS neuropathic pain.
- Antiseizure medications such as Tegretol (carbamazepine) and Neurontin (gabapentin) are commonly used to treat trigeminal neuralgia and dysesthesias.

Other treatments for primary pain include tricyclic antidepressants such as Elavil (amitriptyline) and antispasticity medications such as Lioresal (baclofen) and Zanaflex (tizanidine), especially if muscle spasms are an issue.

Unconventional treatments such as meditation and acupuncture may also be able to help. Years ago, unconventional therapies (also known as "complementary and alternative medicine," or CAM) were often seen as being on the fringe, but they have been increasingly recognized over the past several years.

Secondary Pain

Secondary pain refers to the types of pain that are secondary to the disease process itself, such as muscle stiffness and spasticity. Another common type of secondary pain is musculoskeletal that results from muscle weakness, immobility, and deconditioning. It's important to keep in good physical shape, and this is where a physical therapist, orthopedist, or personal trainer comes in. Talk to your doctor about these types of pain to decide which specialist will benefit you the most. He may also suggest over-the-counter analgesics, such as Motrin (ibuprofen) or Tylenol (acetaminophen).

A Word about Walking

While most people diagnosed with MS will retain their mobility during the course of the disease, two-thirds eventually need some kind of mobility device, whether it's a walker or a cane or a scooter.

Muscle weakness is the most common cause for gait disturbances (difficulty with walking) and can cause problems such as foot drag, toe drop, and other abnormalities. Walking may also be impaired by other MS symptoms, such as lack of coordination, fatigue, spasticity, dizziness, sensory changes, and vertigo. Because so many different factors can sabotage your ability to walk effectively, it's important to pinpoint the cause. Tools such as exercise, physical therapy, medications, and assistive devices can make a big difference. Each person must have his walking difficulties evaluated by a trained health care professional.

Assistive Devices

There are a variety of assistive devices that can help people manage the symptoms of MS, and once folks get past the psychological barriers to using them, they find an increased sense of freedom and opportunity. An assistive device is a tool or a product that makes certain functions easier to perform. An occupational or physical therapist can evaluate your needs and prescribe these devices for you. Here's a list of some tools you might find useful:

- **Orthotics.** These are lightweight inserts worn inside the shoes that can be used to increase stability and decrease fatigue. They also help with spasticity in the foot as well as bracing the foot when walking.
- **Leg braces.** Weakness of the leg muscles can make it difficult to walk up and down the stairs, get up from a chair, or walk. An ankle-foot orthosis (AFO) can help address this issue. The ankle brace stabilizes the ankle if there is weakness in the foot. It fits into an ordinary shoe and prevents the toes from dragging.
- **Canes.** If one leg is weaker than the other, a cane may be your most useful tool. They also help to improve balance. The canes today are not your grandfather's canes. They have models to fit every personality and mood.
- **Walkers.** If there is significant leg weakness, walkers are extremely useful tools, providing balance and stability. Wheels or platforms can also be added.
- **Scooters and wheelchairs.** Technology has helped these devices grow into functional, sleek, and efficient tools for full- or part-time users. Wheelchairs are usually recommended for folks who have excessive fatigue or unsteadiness, or are prone to falling, but others use them on a part-time basis to

conserve energy and stamina. A good resource to help you familiarize yourself with these devices is *www.abledata.com*.

There are thousands of other products on the market to assist in making your life a little easier. From hand-held shower heads to special writing utensils, these devices are there to help you find shortcuts for routine activities so you can better manage your symptoms.

CHAPTER 10

Cognitive Challenges and Mood Changes

COGNITION REFERS TO a whole range of different intellectual processes your brain undertakes to perform tasks and keep you functioning. It incorporates your ability to think, remember, concentrate, and reason. People with MS are sometimes disturbed to learn that along with the physical challenges of MS, cognitive challenges can present themselves as well. While the symptoms are seen in about half of the MS population, only small percentages have cognitive problems severe enough to cause significant changes in their daily lives.

Cognitive Changes

MS may affect cognitive function for several reasons, but the most pervasive is thought to be damage to the nerve cells ("axonal injury"). Stress, anxiety, fatigue, depression, and medication side effects (the indirect effects of the disease process) can also play a role in cognitive dysfunction.

While people who have had MS for a long period of time seem to be more prone to these problems, cognitive dysfunction can be seen early in the disease and have an impact at home or work. Even mild symptoms can be troubling, especially if they interfere with the important tasks of daily living. In fact, people with MS are more likely to leave the work force because of cognitive symptoms and fatigue.

It's important to have any cognitive problems evaluated early on so you can develop a treatment plan with members of your health care team. The following problems seem to be the most common.

Memory Loss

Memory loss is more likely than other problems to be overlooked and misunderstood. But memory problems are the most common type of cognitive dysfunction in MS and can occur at any time during the disease. Recent memory is most often affected by MS. Recent memory refers to newly learned information, such as a person's name or a telephone number. It also includes things you are trying to remember for the future, such as stopping at the store on your way home from work.

Essential

It is important to note that memory loss does not necessarily indicate diminished intelligence or the ability to learn. The brain may simply need more time to recall information from memory or to learn new information. Taking more time to think and having a supportive atmosphere can help solve these challenges.

Forgetting names, losing or misplacing things, and forgetting what you were just doing are all symptoms of memory loss, although it's safe to say everyone experiences these moments from time to time. (Later this chapter will discuss ways to evaluate your cognitive difficulties and learn when to seek help.) Other common cognitive problems may include the following:

- **Attention and concentration.** For many people with MS, maintaining concentration and attention for single tasks is easier than having to focus on several things at once or having to multitask. Folks who have problems with concentration may find it easier to work on just one thing at a time in a quiet environment.
- **Visual spatial skills.** People with MS may have problems perceiving or recognizing objects or orienting themselves. This can interfere with activities such as reading maps or looking at diagrams or charts. It can also make driving difficult.
- **Problem solving.** When confronted with a problem, people with cognitive dysfunction may have difficulty coming up with a solution, or they choose the same solution over and over instead of generating a new one.
- **Language.** The types of language problems most often seen in MS are related to fluency—finding the right words to use when speaking, or using the wrong word.
- **Processing speed.** When processing speed is impaired, a person may have difficulty processing incoming information; they experience a "slowing down" in their brain or a lag in their thoughts.
- **Cognitive fatigue.** Studies show that people with MS can get fatigued when doing challenging work over a long period of time. Some people call it "brain fog." A timeout or a quick break is often helpful in resolving this type of fatigue.
- **Planning and organizing abilities.** People with cognitive difficulties may find it hard to plan or organize.

Research has shown that there are some general tendencies when it comes to cognitive difficulties. Firstly, there is little or no relationship between duration of MS and the severity of cognitive changes. In other words, just because you've had MS for twenty years doesn't mean that you are more likely to experience cognitive symptoms.

People with a progressive form of the disease are at a slightly greater risk of having cognitive problems. Although it's not inevitable, cognitive changes can progress like other symptoms. They can also improve or stay the same.

Fact

Recent studies have shown that about half of all people with MS show no evidence of cognitive dysfunction. About 40 percent have mild dysfunction while 5 to 10 percent have moderate to severe impairments. This means that nine out of ten people with MS are free of severe cognitive difficulties.

Finding Help

If you suspect you might be experiencing cognitive changes, the first thing to do is get in to see your doctor and discuss your concerns. Since so many of these symptoms happen to everyone on occasion, how do you decide if you need help?

The general rule of thumb is to seek an expert opinion when anything that's going on with your life causes you concern. You might say "Geez, I notice I've been doing that a lot lately," or "My bad memory seems to be interfering with my work." If the problem is more subtle, here are some clues that you may need an evaluation:

- You can't explain why things seem more complicated lately at work or at home.
- You notice your memory is failing you several times a day, or more than is normal for you.
- Others have noticed a change in your performance at work or at home and you've eliminated the usual suspects, such as stress or depression.
- You just feel different, perhaps foggy or mentally drained.

The first signs of cognitive dysfunction may be subtle. Often, the family becomes aware of the problem first, noticing changes in behavior or personal habits. Discussing the problem is important, as coping and management strategies can help reduce stress and limit the impact of the symptom. Education, understanding, and acknowledgement play important roles in the social support system on the part of the person with MS.

Three different types of health professionals are able to evaluate cognitive problems: neuropsychologists, speech/language pathologists, or occupational therapists. Your best bet is to ask your neurologist for a recommendation. Whom you seek help from may largely depend on what types of professionals are available in your area. Each uses a different method to assess your difficulties but all three can be effective in diagnosing and measuring cognitive dysfunction.

The Cognitive Evaluation

The gold standard for measuring cognitive function in multiple sclerosis is a full battery of cognitive tests, which include a series of verbal and pencil and paper tests. The testing is usually done by a neuropsychologist, preferably one that has specific training and experience with MS. Their goal is to evaluate if—and how much— cognitive impairment is affecting your daily life.

Your neurologist may give you a brief test in his office to screen for potential problems (He may ask you to count backward by four starting at number twenty-eight, for example). But the full battery of tests will be done in a neuropsychologist's office and may take six to eight hours to complete (sometimes it will be spread out over a few days to minimize fatigue). The test is very costly, so be sure to contact your insurance company before you schedule an appointment to make sure you're covered.

Neuropsychological testing has come quite a long way in the last decade, and tests today are considered to be highly accurate, providing very specific data on a patient's cognitive functioning. The tests cover the range of mental processes from simple motor performance to complex reasoning and problem solving. Many people report leaving the neuropsychological test feeling a little drained, to say the least.

The results of your test will be compared to those of the general population in your age bracket. The test evaluates the specific cognitive problems you might be having and your remaining strengths. Assessing your strengths will allow your specialist to recommend ways to compensate for any deficits you are facing. If your problem, for example, is with short-term memory, you can develop strategies to cope, such as writing things down or buying an electronic device to record daily tasks or reminders. If your problems are caused by difficulty concentrating, you can develop strategies to reduce distractions, such as moving your office to a quieter section of your office building. Your strengths will help you compensate for your weaknesses.

Alert

Unless your doctor is on the lookout for cognition problems, they can be easily missed. You may want to ask him specifically about screening tests for thinking problems.

Cognitive problems can be hard on self esteem. Many people feel a sense of self-doubt when they can't remember things or when they feel they aren't functioning at a peak level. Neuropsychological testing can often be a step toward resolving some of these feelings by letting you know there's a sound reason for your difficulties. It may also relieve the concern of your family members and loved ones.

Treatment Options

It has taken a long time for the medical community to recognize cognitive dysfunction in MS, a frustrating reality for many people who felt their concerns and complaints were ignored. Thankfully, researchers and clinicians have changed their views about cognition in MS and the result has been new strategies and treatment options.

Drug Therapies

There are currently two options when it comes to drug therapy for the treatment of cognitive symptoms. Some studies have shown that Aricept (donepezil) may provide some improvement for memory-related problems. Aricept is an FDA-approved drug prescribed for Alzheimer's disease. However, remember that Alzheimer's and cognitive dysfunction in MS are not related; they are different diseases.

Your second option is the disease-modifying therapies. They've been shown to reduce the number and severity of MS attacks. Starting Avonex, Betaseron, Copaxone, or Rebif early may help to prevent cognitive dysfunction.

Cognitive Rehabilitation

The goal of cognitive rehabilitation therapy is to help an individual acquire the highest level of cognitive functioning possible. This is accomplished through treatment programs that focus on retraining strategies and teach skills that help individuals compensate.

Cognitive retraining employs two different strategies. The first, restoration, involves restoring cognitive skills in the same way you might rebuild a weakened muscle. Exercises, some done with computer programs, can help build cognitive skills such as attention, concentration, memory, and organization.

The second component of cognitive retraining, compensation, involves learning to use strategies and tools to cope with weaker areas. Strategies are designed for each patient that use her areas of strength to compensate for her weakened abilities. Learning to use these tools not only compensates for impaired ability, but may help to rebuild the skill itself. For example, regularly using a checklist may actually improve attention skills. Rehabilitation programs usually use a combination of restoration and compensatory techniques.

Toolbox for Cognitive Challenges

There are some good ways to compensate for cognitive difficulties at home, ranging from keeping lists to tactics used for problem solving.

Implementing changes in your life can be frustrating, but repeated use of these tips can help you form healthy habits.

Memory

Write things down! Be sure to include the "who, what, where, when, and why" so your notes contain the critical data that you need. Use a daily planner to keep track of all of your information. Use a pill-box with slots for every day of the week to keep track of your medication. Check out electronic gadgets, such as mini tape recorders, to assist you if note taking is challenging.

Problem Solving

Come up with several different strategies for any given situation and list the pros and the cons of each solution. Consider asking someone else for their input. Since problem-solving skills are often slower in individuals who are experiencing cognitive difficulties, taking your time and thinking things through can help you get past the frustration.

Organization

Make a checklist of tasks, breaking down larger tasks into smaller parts. Get all of the supplies you'll need and organize them in your workspace. Plan your day early in the morning. Remember to prioritize and pace yourself. Work on more demanding tasks when your energy level is higher.

Attention

Try to avoid fatigue by taking mental breaks. Keep yourself on task by asking yourself if you are doing what you'd planned to be doing right now. Keep the television and radio off to minimize distractions.

The trick to cognitive retraining is your willingness to learn and your flexibility to integrate new strategies. Being patient with yourself, asking for help, and practicing new skills will facilitate your success.

Mood Swings and Emotional Challenges

Most people have experienced mood swings at some point in their life and they can usually pinpoint the cause; hormonal changes, stress, and fatigue are examples. Mood swings and uncontrolled emotion in MS, however, tend to be more common than in the general population. Those who deal with these challenges describe symptoms that range from angry outbursts to uncontrollable laughing and crying and inappropriate giddiness. These problems are not the same as the reaction you may have to a new MS diagnosis, for instance, where an emotional response (such as, sadness) is a normal part of the acceptance process.

Involuntary Emotional Expressive Disorder (IEED)

What this mouthful means in a nutshell is this: IEED is a disorder that causes sudden and unpredictable episodes of laughing, crying, or other emotional displays. No one is really sure what causes this neurologic disorder, but it is thought that lesions in the frontal lobe (which keeps emotion in check) compromise its ability to function properly. This damage can disrupt brain signaling, causing a short circuit that triggers the episodes. About 10 percent of the MS population is affected by IEED, but it is most often seen in those who have progressive disease and significant cognitive changes.

Essential

It is important to clarify the cause of emotional problems because a diagnosis will determine the course of treatment. IEED should be separated from other problems, such as depression. Patients who experience these episodes can often be embarrassed by them and avoid social contact, so early recognition and management is important to maintaining a healthy life.

Treatment

Treatment is still evolving, but the same drugs used to treat depression are often effective in IEED, such as Elavil (amitriptyline) or Prozac (fluoxetine). Dextromethorphan, a component of some cough syrup, is being studied to treat patients who have IEED.

Handling Mood Swings

Medications and counseling are effective treatment strategies for mood swings, but there are other ways to help you cope.

Studies show that regular exercise can help improve mood and even help you sleep better. Exercising twenty minutes a day, three times a week can help you to focus your energy and leave your emotions behind for a while.

Using your support network to talk things out can also be beneficial, especially with others who are experiencing some of the same things that you are. And talk to your doctor if your mood swings aren't improving despite your interventions.

There's nothing like a whole lot of stress (or even a little) to exacerbate your symptoms, including mood swings. Find ways to relax, such as reading or taking a walk. You might want to look into some other approaches, such as yoga and meditation.

Controlling Depression

It is important for people with MS to be on the lookout for depression—not just those days when you're singing the blues, but the sort of depression that interferes with your daily activities. Depression can pack a big punch and can cause difficulties with relationships, work, and family, not to mention all the joy it can steal from your life.

Depression is very common in people with multiple sclerosis. In fact, significant depression occurs in about half of all people with MS at some point during their illness. As a result, it's important to recognize the signs.

When feelings of sadness become intense and last for long periods of time, it's a good sign that you may be depressed. Other signs and symptoms include:

- Sustained lack of energy
- Loss of interest in hobbies or activities
- Feelings of hopelessness and worthlessness
- Difficulty concentrating
- Excessive sleeping or inability to stay or fall asleep
- Decreased sex drive
- Weight loss or weight gain
- Thoughts of death or suicide

You may have noticed that many of the signs of depression are also symptoms of MS. That's why talking to your doctor is so important—it can be tricky to sort out what is really going on. You should also discuss your medications with your health care provider to see if any of your meds are affecting your mood. Possible culprits are the interferon therapies (Avonex, Betaseron, and Rebif) and corticosteroids.

Question

What causes depression in MS?
MS may destroy the insulating myelin that surrounds nerves that transmit signals affecting mood. People with MS may also feel depressed about the challenges brought on by the disease. In addition, some of the drugs used to treat MS can cause depression.

Treatment

Trying to "get over" depression by yourself isn't realistic. Depression is a serious illness that requires immediate attention and careful monitoring by a physician or mental health professional—

preferably one who has experience with the depression caused by MS. The best way to find a health professional who has experience with MS is to ask your neurologist or the physician who is taking care of your MS for a referral. You can also contact the main office or your local chapter of the NMSS at 1-800-FIGHT-MS for the names of health professionals experienced with both depression and MS in your area.

Alert

The diagnosis of depression is made by observation and conversation, since there aren't any medical tests—like a blood test—to aid in diagnosis. Your doctor will ask you a series of questions about your family history, your symptoms, drug and alcohol abuse, and whether you have thoughts of suicide. It is important that you answer these questions honestly so your doctor can figure out the best treatment plan for you.

A combination of psychotherapy and medication is often the most effective approach for treating depression. The most common types of medication include:

Selective Serotonin Reuptake Inhibiters (SSRIs)
Drugs such as Prozac (fluoxetine), Zoloft (sertraline), Celexa (citalopram), and Paxil (paroxetine), are a few of the drugs among the SSRIs that are used to treat depression and anxiety disorders. Potential side effects differ for each drug.

Selective Serotonin and Norepinephrine Reuptake Inhibitors (SSNRI)
Studies have shown that this newer class of drugs is effective in treating depressive disorder. These drugs include Effexor (venlafaxine hydrochloride) and Cymbalta (duloxetine hydrochloride).

Tricyclic Antidepressants

This older class of drugs is used less frequently because these drugs generally have more side effects and may be less effective than the SSRIs and SSNRIs.

Essential

Research indicates that the most effective treatment for depression may be a combination of treatment with antidepressant medications and "talk therapy" or psychotherapy. Psychiatrists, clinical psychologists, and social workers may provide psychotherapy. Your local MS Society chapter may be able to give you a list of MS support groups in your area or mental health professionals experienced in working with people with MS.

It's important to be educated about the cognitive difficulties in MS. You want to be on the lookout for signs of depression or problems with memory. But it's also important to keep a healthy perspective. Most people with MS do not face significant cognitive impairment. And now that cognitive dysfunction has been accepted as a valid symptom in the MS medical community, new treatments and coping strategies are on the horizon. As with any challenge in multiple sclerosis, it's important to be educated while keeping an optimistic and hopeful attitude.

CHAPTER 11

Complementary and Alternative Therapy

COMPLEMENTARY AND ALTERNATIVE medicine (CAM) has become increasingly popular in Western society over the past few decades. Those that pursue CAM are interested in treating illnesses or maintaining or achieving optimum health. It is a field that is constantly evolving, and some of its basic treatments (such as exercise or the benefits of vitamins) are no longer considered "alternative," but are accepted as basic tenets in maintaining health.

What Is CAM?

The term *unconventional therapy* is used to describe any medical treatment or intervention that is not generally taught in medical schools or generally available at hospitals. The term *complementary and alternative medicine (CAM)* is also used to describe these therapies. Complementary medicine indicates unconventional therapies that are used in conjunction with conventional medicine, while alternative medicine refers to unconventional therapies that are used instead of conventional medicine. CAM encompasses a variety of disciplines that range from diet and exercise to mind-body approaches and lifestyle changes. Examples include acupuncture, yoga, aromatherapy, relaxation, herbal remedies, and massage.

Most people with MS choose to use complementary therapy to treat their MS, which means they adhere to a routine of conventional medicines (interferon therapy, for example) along with some form of unconventional intervention, such as practicing yoga or taking daily supplements. Before you consider any therapy—unconventional or otherwise—it's always important to discuss your options with your health care team. Since many forms of CAM are unregulated, it is all too common to find that the claims of some products or services are false. This means that you might be out of pocket whatever you spent on the product or service. In rare instances, it can also be dangerous to your health.

Types of CAM

The National Institute of Health divides CAM into different categories:

- Mind-body medicine incorporates various techniques to enhance the mind's capacity to affect a person's health. Techniques in this category include prayer and meditation.
- Biologically based practices in CAM refer generally to diets and dietary supplements, such as vitamins, minerals, and herbs.
- Manipulative and body-based systems are based on the manipulation or movement of one or more body parts, such as massage or chiropractic manipulation.
- Energy medicine is divided into two parts: Biofield therapies affect energy fields that are thought to exist in the human body. Bioelectromagnetic-based therapy uses electromagnetic fields and includes the use of magnets.
- Whole medical systems includes therapies from traditional Chinese medicine and the Indian practice of Ayurveda.

Choosing Wisely

The established medical community often casts a somewhat wary eye on CAM. One concern is that there is limited or no scientific evidence about the safety and effectiveness of some CAM interventions. Conventional drugs are tested for safety and effectiveness by clinically controlled scientific studies, while many CAM approaches have not been tested in such a rigorous way. Within conventional medicine, treatments cannot be claimed to be beneficial or safe unless this has been demonstrated through rigorous testing. The FDA has a set of standards and documentation requirements that prove a treatment has reasonable risks and benefits.

Essential

For more information, the National Center for Complementary and Alternative Medicine (NCCAM), can help you get up to speed on CAM therapies and products. Check out their website at *www.nccam.nih.gov.* The Office of Dietary Supplements, is also a great resource. Visit their website at *www.ods.od.nih.gov.* Furthermore, the book *Complementary and Alternative Medicine for Multiple Sclerosis* provides authoritative information.

Unlike conventional medicine, most CAM therapies have not been subjected to rigorous FDA standards, so it's important to be an educated consumer. Keeping that in mind, CAM can be an important part of your treatment plan, as it has been reported to help people with MS treat some of their symptoms. Being a smart CAM consumer requires you to be resourceful and do some digging. Here are some tips to help you get started:

- Be an informed consumer. Find out what scientific studies have been done on the safety and effectiveness of the CAM treatment in which you are interested.

- Check with your doctor before making decisions about your treatment or care.
- Be wary of superlatives, such as "miracle cure!" Right now, there is no known cure for MS, so be cautious of any treatment or product that claims it can cure you.
- Know the risks. Is there anyone for whom the therapy is not recommended? Someone who is pregnant, for instance, or has diabetes?
- Make sure the practitioner has the appropriate credentials or licenses to practice.
- Check out the practice or therapy you are interested in by using more than one source. Research websites created by major medical centers, universities, and government agencies. They are often the most credible.
- Search for the most recent information you can find. Reputable websites cite a date for each article they post.
- Stay away from research that doesn't clearly distinguish between scientific evidence and advertisements.
- Be clear about what the treatment involves.
- Understand the costs involved.

Unfortunately, scammers have perfected ways to convince you that their therapy is best. The FDA recommends that you watch out for red-flag words such as "satisfaction guaranteed," "miracle cures," or "new discovery." If the product were in fact a cure, it would be widely reported in the media and your doctor would recommend it.

Pseudomedical jargon should also send up a red flag. Terms such as "purify," "detoxify," and "energize" may sound impressive and may even have an element of truth, but they're often used to cover up a lack of proven efficacy.

If a manufacturer claims that the product can treat a wide range of symptoms, or cure or prevent a number of diseases, be prepared to scrutinize. No single product can do all this.

Anecdotal evidence can sound impressive, but testimonials are no substitute for solid scientific documentation. If the product is scientifically sound, it's actually to the manufacturer's advantage to promote the scientific evidence.

Understanding Studies

You will come across all kinds of studies as you research MS treatments, CAM interventions, and the like. Here's the skinny on the difference between clinical, randomized, and double-blind studies:

- *Clinical studies* involve human beings and not animals. (Generally, they follow studies that demonstrate the safety and effectiveness of the treatment in animals in a laboratory setting.)
- In *randomized* studies, human participants are usually divided into groups. One group receives the treatment under study, and another (the control group) receives the standard treatment, no treatment, or a placebo (an inactive substance). The participants are assigned to the groups on a random basis.
- In *double-blind* studies, neither the research participants nor the researchers know which treatment is being administered to whom.

One or two small studies, whether the results are positive or negative, usually aren't enough to make a definite decision about whether to use or approve a specific treatment. Unfortunately, there are a limited number of quality studies on many CAM treatments. Keep in mind that while solid research studies are the best way to evaluate whether a treatment is safe and effective, a lack of solid evidence doesn't always mean that these treatments don't work—but it does mean that they haven't been proven.

Fact

In the United States, 36 percent of adults are using some form of CAM. When megavitamin therapy and prayer (specifically for health reasons) are included in the definition of CAM, that number rises to 62 percent. The survey found that most people use CAM along with conventional medicine rather than in place of conventional medicine.

CAM Therapies for MS

CAM use in the treatment of MS appears to be greater than that of the general population. In several studies that looked at people from various countries throughout the world, it was found that one-half to three-quarters of the people studied used some form of unconventional medicine in conjunction with conventional medicine. Special diets, dietary supplements, prayer and spirituality, chiropractic medicine, and massage topped the list as the most commonly used CAM therapies.

Alert

It is important to remember that of all the conventional and unconventional therapies used in the treatment of MS, only the interferons, and glatiramer acetate, mitoxantrone, and natalizumab (Tysabri) have evidence that they can effectively alter the course of the disease. There are currently no CAM therapies that have a similar level of evidence to support their use as disease-modifying therapies.

It is also important to determine when to consider the use of CAM. Finding unconventional therapies for mild fatigue or muscle stiffness is reasonable, but there are certain situations, such as severe pain or disabling weakness, in which using CAM exclusively is inappropriate.

Also keep in mind that there are quite a few misconceptions about dietary supplements, which include vitamins, minerals, and herbs. Many of these products claim to have no side effects, which is not true. Some supplements, especially herbs, are similar to medications and contain chemicals that may cause side effects. Even so-called natural products can be toxic, such as poisonous mushrooms or mercury. Also note that the quality of supplements varies widely.

Fact

The thoughtful use of CAM can indeed provide benefits. A Canadian study that included nearly 700 subjects with MS showed that 72 percent reported positive results from CAM treatments. In this study, patients regarded massage therapy and acupuncture as particularly beneficial. Even though some reports of success from CAM are not based on rigorous studies, it is clear that people with MS regard these therapies as valuable additions to conventional management therapies.

Vitamins, Minerals, and Herbs

A vitamin is a small molecule that your body needs to carry out specific biological processes. Since your body has no way to create vitamins itself, it relies on the food that you eat (except for vitamin D, which needs the sun to synthesize the vitamin). Your body uses the vitamins in unique ways. For example, vitamin A produces retinol that in turn is used by the rods and the cones in your eyes to sense light.

Following are the dietary supplements most commonly used by people with MS.

Antioxidants

Vitamins A, C, and E are known antioxidants, and although research is limited, some studies suggest they may be helpful in reducing the effects of MS. Keep in mind that some antioxidants could potentially worsen the disease, as they've been shown to activate immune cells that are already overly active. Further studies are currently under way. It's best to talk to your doctor before taking antioxidants.

Vitamin D and Calcium

Vitamin D helps maintain healthy bones by increasing the absorption of calcium and helps to prevent osteoporosis. People with MS have an increased risk of developing osteoporosis, so the use of these vitamins—in regular doses—may be beneficial. Studies are under way to determine if vitamin D plays a role in the development of MS. Researchers are searching for a connection between lack of vitamin D and the prevalence of MS in regions where sunlight is scarce.

Vitamin B12

This vitamin helps to promote normal CNS function, but there doesn't seem to be any benefit in taking this vitamin to people whose B_{12} levels are normal. A small subset of people with MS have B_{12} deficiency and they should be treated with supplements or monthly injections.

Valerian

Some studies show that valerian may be beneficial in treating insomnia but its use in treating spasticity and anxiety has not been evaluated extensively by research.

Vitamin C

This vitamin is often used for the prevention or treatment of urinary tract infections, though studies have not validated this claim.

Ginkgo Biloba

Ginkgo biloba is a popular herb that has been extensively studied. While there is little clinical evidence to support claims that it is beneficial for treating MS itself, a few studies have found it improved cognitive function.

Echinacea

Immune-stimulating dietary supplements can pose a risk to people with MS because they activate the immune system. Other herbs in this category include Asian and Siberian ginseng, cat's claw, stinging nettle, garlic, mistletoe, saw palmetto, and shiitake mushrooms. Consult with your doctor about taking echinacea.

Cranberry

Cranberry may be effective for preventing urinary tract infections in women with normal bladder function but should not be used to treat UTIs.

St. John's Wort

This supplement may be effective for treating mild to moderate depression, although it's important not to diagnose and treat depression on your own. St. John's wort may also interact with other medications you may be taking, so it's important to confer with your health care provider

Other CAM Interventions

People with MS have used other interventions with varying degrees of success. They include:

Bee Venom Therapy

Apitherapy (using bee stings or bee products medicinally) has been used to treat medical conditions since ancient times. Studies of bee venom therapy in people with MS and in an animal model of MS found it to be ineffective. Some people may have severe allergic reactions to bee venom.

Marijuana

While quite a bit of attention has been focused on the use of marijuana for medicinal purposes, research is still under way and the jury is still out. There have been many anecdotal reports of the success of cannabis in treating MS symptoms, particularly spasticity. However, there is little rigorous scientific evidence that the drug works, although research is currently under way. Cannabis is still illegal in many states and countries, although some states grant legal permission to dispense marijuana for medicinal purposes.

Question

What are the side effects of using marijuana as a CAM therapy?
The results of one study showed that people with MS who smoke marijuana are more likely to have memory and emotional problems. The 2007 study was conducted by researchers at the University of Toronto. The study found marijuana smokers performed 50 percent slower on tests of information processing speed compared to MS patients who did not smoke marijuana. There was also a significant association between smoking marijuana and emotional problems such as depression and anxiety.

Cooling Therapy

This therapy involves the use of cooling devices that are designed to remove excess heat from the body. These devices come in various forms, including wet scarves tied around the neck, vests filled with frozen packets, and hoods and vests that attach to cooling pumps. The purpose of this therapy is to help speed nerve conduction in people with MS. Studies indicate that cooling may help ease various MS symptoms including fatigue, impaired visual function, weakness, and cognitive difficulties.

Acupuncture

Acupuncture is part of traditional Chinese medicine and involves the use of thin needles that are inserted in strategic points on the body to alter the body's energy flow. Limited studies suggest that acupuncture may provide relief from anxiety, weakness, pain, dizziness, and depression.

Chiropractic Medicine

Chiropractic medicine is based on the principle that spinal joint misalignments interfere with the nervous system and can thereby result in many different diseases. Currently, there is no established evidence that chiropractic therapy is beneficial for MS attacks or for altering the course of the disease.

Dental Amalgam Removal

Removal of the silver-colored fillings used to fill cavities is proposed as a treatment for MS. It is based on the theory that the mercury contained within the fillings is toxic to the body's immune system or nervous system. Despite some anecdotal reports on the benefits of this rather expensive procedure, there is no strong evidence that amalgam removal improves the course of MS.

Diets

Special diets have received a lot of press in the CAM arena because of anecdotal reports from various people with MS who have claimed significant benefits from various diets.

Fact

The Swank diet, devised and championed by Dr. Roy Swank in 1948, advocates a dietary approach low in saturated fats for the management of multiple sclerosis. Swank's research on 144 patients over a thirty-four year period showed that those who followed the diet did not show any significant deterioration of their condition. Swank's study did not include a placebo-treated group and thus was not rigorous enough to allow definitive conclusions.

Other studies have shown that diets low in saturated fats and high in polyunsaturated fatty acids (PUFAs) may have a therapeutic effect in MS. Supplementation with omega-6 fatty acids and omega-3 fatty acids has been well tolerated in clinical trials and may have some benefit. If this approach is used, it should be used in conjunction with, *not instead of*, conventional disease-modifying therapies.

Guided Imagery and Relaxation

To date, one small study found that guided imagery reduced anxiety in people with MS. In guided imagery, an individual creates mental images that purportedly have specific effects on the mind and body.

Massage

Massage is believed to improve the circulation of blood and lymph, creating better oxygen flow and the removal of harmful toxins. It may also decrease muscle stiffness and release endorphins, which are the body's natural pain-relieving chemicals. Limited studies show that massage may be beneficial in MS, improving mood and reducing spasticity.

Magnets and Electromagnetic Therapy

Some studies suggest that magnetic therapy with magnetic fields may be beneficial for certain symptoms in MS, including spasticity and bladder problems. Further study in this area is needed. Pregnant women and people with electronic medical implants should consult their physicians before using these devices.

Biofeedback

Biofeedback therapy uses monitoring equipment to translate different bodily reactions into pictures or sounds. Several studies (not conducted on people with MS) have shown biofeedback to be potentially beneficial for spasticity, pain, depression, reduced cognitive functioning, and other disorders common to MS.

Chelation Therapy

This type of therapy uses chemicals (whether by ingestion or intravenously) that bind to metals in the blood. There is no evidence that chelation is useful in treating multiple sclerosis, although it is useful in treating cases of heavy-metal toxicity.

The Spiritual Approach

Some types of CAM tap into the spiritual side of life, with prayer and meditation as the backdrop. Spiritual-based CAM approaches include:

- **Prayer.** According to some surveys, prayer is the most frequently used form of CAM in the United States. Scientists are increasingly attempting to measure the effect of prayer on patients' health. Additional studies are needed, with clear descriptions of prayer techniques and well-defined health outcomes.
- **Yoga.** There are limited studies of yoga's effects on MS. One large, well-designed study found that yoga was helpful for decreasing fatigue. Limited reports indicate that it may also help relieve pain and anxiety. In the Hindu tradition, yoga is said to increase the stores of vital energy.
- **Tai chi.** This therapy is a component of traditional Chinese medicine and combines meditation with physical exercise. Tai chi is said to create emotional balance by uniting the two life-energy forces of yin and yang. In one small study, symptom improvement in people with MS was noted, particularly in muscle stiffness.
- **Aromatherapy.** This therapy involves treating conditions by the use of essential oils that are purported to promote an increase of energy and relaxation. It may be beneficial for anxiety and depression, but further study is needed.

When used to complement traditional treatment, the thoughtful use of CAM can be an important part of MS management. Since research and regulation on CAM therapies is still somewhat lax, it is important to choose wisely and be cautious. Remember to discuss your ideas with your MS specialist before trying something new.

CHAPTER 12

Stress and MS

IT WASN'T LONG ago that science insisted stress had little influence on MS—or, for that matter, on health in general. Despite anecdotal evidence from patients that stress seemed to exacerbate their MS symptoms, it wasn't generally recognized as an influencing factor in the disease. The jury is still out on whether it plays a definitive role in causing exacerbations, but some studies indicate there may be a relationship between stress and the onset of MS. A recent Dutch study found that ongoing stressful life conditions may make MS symptoms worse.

The Science Behind Stress

Stress has played an important role in the development of man. The fight-or-flight reaction is humankind's primitive and automatic response that prepares the body to flee from a perceived attack or threat to survival. When we experience stress, a bodily reaction is triggered, bypassing our logical mind.

The parasympathetic system, regulated by the brain, calms the body while the sympathetic system prepares the body for the fight-or-flight reaction. This "hard-wired" response is both psychological and physical in nature and causes your heart to beat faster, your muscles to tense, your palms to sweat, and your breathing rate and blood pressure to increase. And it's not just physical threats that cause this response: psychological trauma can also inflame the emotional centers of the brain, causing a constant outflow of the fight-or-flight reaction. This physiological activity may cause your symptoms to act up, too.

These days, there aren't a lot of physical stressors such as saber-toothed tigers that threaten you. Today's stressors are psychological in nature: deadlines at work, rush-hour traffic, and cancelled flights. Having MS in itself is a stressor. And since you can't really "run" anywhere, you are faced with having to learn how to handle stress within the contours of your life.

 Alert

> Chronic stress isn't good for anyone, and you might be worried that it isn't good for MS either. But having MS is stressful in itself, even without the rest of the outside stressors most people contend with. So, while stress may be hard for you to avoid, the trick is to learn how to manage it successfully and minimize its effects on your health and well-being.

Stress management can be complicated; people contend with different types of stress on a daily basis and each one has its own characteristics, duration, and treatment. Here's a look at the three types of stress:

- **Acute stress.** This is the most common form of stress and it hails from the everyday pressures and demands of life. In other words, it's a reality all people deal with. Since it's part of the fight-or-flight reaction, acute stress is okay in small doses. It's short-term, too, so for the most part it doesn't have the ability to cause significant damage that long-term stress does.

- **Episodic acute stress.** Someone suffering from this form of stress is living a busy, chaotic life and tends to be irritable, tense, and short on patience. "Worry warts" and type A personalities tend to suffer from episodic acute stress. Symptoms include headaches, hypertension, chest pain, and heart disease.
- **Chronic stress.** This type of stress wears you down, day after day, year after year. It is caused by being exposed to long-term stressors such as unhappy marriages or careers. If an individual sees no hope in improving his situation, he often gives up looking for solutions. Chronic stress can lead to depression and a host of physical ailments, such as heart disease.

Knowing the different types of stress is important. Some stress can motivate you to reach a deadline, while other types can wreak havoc on your life. Unfortunately, your body doesn't make the distinction between physical or psychological stress, so facing a medical test or a screaming toddler can both put you into overdrive. That's because the fight-or-flight reaction kicks in to help you cope with the perceived threat. When the demands of life exceed your ability to cope, stress can harm your physical and mental well-being.

The Symptoms of Stress

To get a good handle on it, you'll have to identify your own signs of stress. Stress affects the mind, body, and behavior in different ways, so the symptoms vary between people. Some folks will get a backache, others will feel sick to their stomach, and still others will exhibit emotional problems. Stress can even change the way you behave and think. Here are a few of the many symptoms of stress:

- Inability to concentrate
- Memory problems
- Moodiness

- Short temper
- Restlessness
- Feeling overwhelmed
- Muscle tension or stiffness
- Weight loss or weight gain
- Frequent colds
- Sleeping too much or too little
- Nervous habits

You may have noticed that some of these symptoms overlap MS symptoms, such as muscle tension or stiffness, inability to concentrate, and memory problems. That makes it all the more important that you identify your stressors so you can distinguish them from MS symptoms that need your attention. These days, people have a tendency to blame everything on stress. Conversely, some people with MS may blame all of their physical symptoms on MS, even when other things, such as stress or a virus, may be responsible. It's a good thing to see your doctor if you're exhibiting any of the symptoms listed above. She can help figure out what may be causing them.

Identifying Your Stressors

Like everyone else, you probably have a lot of responsibilities and worries—a career, a family, long commutes, a mortgage. And of course, managing MS brings on a whole other slew of concerns and stressors. But here's the reason why you have to get stress under control: The more the stress response is activated, the harder it is to shut off. Even when the crisis is past, your heart rate, stress hormones, and blood pressure remain elevated. This can all take a big toll on your body. Long-term exposure to stress can cause obesity, heart disease, anxiety, and memory problems. Your goal then, is to reduce its impact on your daily life.

What you consider to be stressful is unique to you. Your personality, your social support system, and your temperament are a few of the factors that determine your potential stressors.

📋 **Fact**

> While most people consider negatives—such as a crazy morning commute or a problematic relationship—to be major causes of stress, in truth, anything that causes you to adjust is a potential stressor. Even good things such as getting married or going on a vacation can put you into overdrive. Anything that pushes the limits of your coping skills and resources can result in stress.

Learning how to cope with stress is the key to your well-being. Your best bet is to sit down and make a list of what stresses you out. Note activities that put a strain on your energy and time or trigger anger or anxiety. You may also want to note positive experiences, especially those that give you a sense of well-being or produce a sense of accomplishment. Take a few days or weeks if you need to make this list; it might take some time to identify your triggers. Following are some of the common stressors for people living with MS.

Daily Demands

Battling traffic, doing injections, and medical appointments are some of the typical daily demands of people living with MS. By themselves, they are small upsets, but piled up together they can make for a stressful day. It's imperative to get a handle on your daily stress levels.

- **Learn to pare down your lists.** There's a difference between "should" and "must." Know the difference between them and prioritize your tasks.
- **Say "no."** Identify your limits and stick to them. Adding responsibilities to an already hectic day may guarantee that you're taking on more than you can handle.
- **Delegate.** It's time to get the kids to wash the dishes and help mow the lawn. There are hundreds of ways you can minimize

household chores, including delegating responsibility, hiring others to clean or do yard work, or letting go of perfectionist tendencies.

- **Manage your time.** Time management remains one of the most effective ways to deal with stress. Make a daily schedule and stick with it. Reward yourself at the end of the day for staying calm and focused.
- **Be assertive.** If you're too tired to drive your daughter to the movies, then say so. It isn't easy to teach others to respect your boundaries, but if you're consistent, they'll learn.

A good rule of thumb is to learn to alter stressful situations that you can't avoid. Take the train to work, start a carpool for soccer practice, and buy the birthday cake instead of making one.

Work can also be a source of daily stress. Things such as job satisfaction, a big workload, or feeling as if you're not making the grade can all contribute to a stressful work life. Many people with MS have had to take a good look at their present employment situation and decide whether or not to find a less stressful job. Those who decide to stay with their job cope best by learning stress-management skills.

MS Stress

When it comes to stressors that you cannot change, acceptance is your only alternative. You cannot prevent the death of a loved one, change the content of the evening news, or, unfortunately, change the fact that you have MS. Many things in life are beyond your control, but you have a choice as to how you handle and react to them. Focus on those things you can control.

So, what can you control when it comes to your life and having MS? It's a good thing to think about, because the answers you come up with will largely determine how well you manage your condition.

Staying healthy by eating well and exercising regularly is a good way to control the overall state of your health. You can also agree to focus on the positive things in your life. Education and commitment are also stress relievers. Stay on top of new treatments and therapies and commit to your medication regimen. It's also important to see your specialists on a regular basis.

Question

Can emotional stress affect daily functioning with MS?
It may. Many people with MS report that their chronic symptoms get worse when they're upset, nervous, or feeling unusually stressed. This condition is only temporary and does *not* represent worsening of the disease. Once you have coped with the stress or begin to relax, the symptoms should disappear.

MS stress can also be caused by fear of the unknown, so identifying your fears and facing each and every one of them is a good idea. Reframe your fears by trying to take a positive approach. For example, if one of your fears is that someday you might need a cane, take that fear out and analyze it. What if you do need a cane one day? You might imagine in your mind all of the people in the world who have had to use a cane. Consider that most of those people adjusted to using a cane and lived good lives despite it. Sometimes when people dissect their fears, they find they aren't as scary as they had once imagined them to be. In fact, facing your fears head-on is a good way to take the air out of them. It may be helpful to visualize the worst possible outcome while keeping in mind that most people with MS do not need a wheelchair.

Adapting to the unavoidable things that cause you stress can help you regain a sense of control. See the challenges before you as an opportunity for personal growth—as well as the growth of those around you.

Stress on the Home Front

Familial stress seems to have its own label; it's composed of many different factors, including relationship, environmental, and financial factors. Problems with a spouse, a noisy neighbor, and a broken washing machine can each contribute to the menu of stressors that make up your daily life at home. Careful planning and time management can help. Delegating tasks and learning to be assertive about your needs can also go a long way in helping you to cope. Family relationships can be complicated, so be sure to seek out help if you're having problems getting everyone to agree on a course of action. You may want to get a referral to an individual, couples, or family therapist. Home should be your salvation—the place where you can unwind and enjoy a reprieve from the daily grind of life.

Fact

When it comes to stress, people rate death of a spouse as the most stressful life event, followed by divorce, separation, and spending time in jail. Death of a loved one and illness are next, with marriage, pregnancy, and retirement rounding out the remainder of the list. Notice that even happy events can be considered stressful. Anything that causes change can be a potential stressor.

Emotional Stressors

It probably doesn't come as a big surprise to learn that people can be their own worst enemies. Not all stress is caused by outside factors; we often do a pretty good job of it ourselves. Worrying, low self-esteem, seeking perfection—these are all self-generated types of internal stress. A good way to resolve internal stress is to set up realistic goals and expectations for your life. Since it's often hard to change behaviors, it may be wise to seek out professional help.

Creating a Stress-Management Plan

Once you've identified the stressors in your life, you're on your way to developing a stress-management plan. You'll want to find healthy ways to manage stress and turn them into strategies that become a habitual part of your life. Keep in mind that there are many books, tapes, and classes (check your local hospital) that can help you manage stress, but following are some tips to get you started.

Evaluate Your Coping Strategies

How do you normally cope with stress? Do you reach for a cigarette or a submarine sandwich? There are a myriad of unhealthy coping strategies, including overeating, oversleeping, and drugs. Coping strategies should add to your state of happiness and well-being.

Adopt a Healthy Lifestyle

There is no question that exercise, good nutrition, and sleep habits go a long way in helping you deal with stress. Exercise is a good way to relieve pent-up tension, and eating right keeps enough fuel in your tank to help you manage whatever comes your way. Being tired can aggravate stress and often makes things seem worse than they really are.

Be Good to Yourself

Never underestimate the benefits of nurturing yourself. There is nothing like a long bath after a hard day, a weekend spent fishing with the guys, or a night out with your spouse to put things in perspective. When you don't replenish your internal wells, your spirit dries up and you have little left to give to others. You should do something you enjoy every day, whether it's walking in nature, reading a book, or taking a yoga class. Connecting with others and indulging your sense of humor are also good ways to nurture yourself. *See this as a necessity rather than a luxury.*

Keep a Journal

Writing every day is a good way to transfer stress and hash out your feelings. It will also help you to identify stressors. Look for common patterns or themes and strategize ways to handle things differently. Journaling is a great opportunity for self-discovery.

Stress-Management Techniques

If you haven't caught on yet, exercise and diet are definitely good for a healthy lifestyle. You might be wondering what else you can do to put a lid on stress, once you get the jumping jacks started and the salad dressed. Quite a few of these techniques are mentioned in Chapter 14, but here is a quick look at them for you to contemplate which strategies may be a good fit for you.

Cognitive Behavioral Therapy (CBT)

Studies have shown that CBT can have a long-term effect on one's ability to cope with stress. The participants in one study who received CBT training had significantly reduced stress responses compared with participants who had no training. CBT may be particularly helpful when the source of stress is chronic pain or a chronic illness. CBT strives to teach you to identify and change your response to sources of stress and to find better ways to cope with it. If this type of therapy interests you, find a therapist who specializes in CBT.

Essential

There is no way to directly measure stress, but its effects on the body can be measured. Heart rate, blood pressure, muscle tension, and breathing rates can all indicate what level of stress an individual is experiencing. These symptoms are not always perceptible, however. Biofeedback is a good way to learn how your body reacts to stress.

Relaxation Methods

Stress is a part of modern life; avoiding it completely isn't possible. A certain amount of stress can be found in every workplace and in every home. Learning some simple relaxation methods can help you handle the common stressors of everyday life. When you're in a relaxed state, blood pressure, muscle tension, respiration rate, and pulse rate decrease in your body and emotional strain begins to cease. Here are a few relaxation methods to consider:

- **Imagery.** The idea behind this relaxation technique is to use your imagination to conjure up the most relaxing scene you can think of.
- **Music and relaxation tapes.** If you're too tired to concentrate, listening to calming music or popping in a prepared tape is a passive way to relax.
- **Meditation.** Research has shown that meditation is a good tool for managing stress. The idea behind this technique is to calm your body by focusing the mind for a sustained period of time.
- **Yoga.** This mind-body technique is getting a lot of press these days as studies have shown that it's effective for all sorts of conditions, including chronic stress. Yoga teams deep breathing with stretching, which may create balance in the body.
- **Deep breathing.** Even taking two minutes to do some deep-breathing exercises can relieve stress. Take slow, deep breaths and focus on relieving any tension you feel in your muscles.

It is well known that strong emotional and social support is integral to managing stress. Laboratory studies show that when subjects are subjected to stress, emotional support reduces the usual sharp rise in blood pressure and increased secretion of damaging stress-related hormones. Developing a strong support network isn't just a good idea—it's important to your health.

Putting Your Plan to Use

You've got your yoga mat, Beethoven tapes, and journal, so now what? How do you develop a routine? Everyone knows what can happen to good intentions (dust on the exercise bike in the basement; running shoes still in the box). Research shows it takes about thirty days to develop a habit, so a good way to psych yourself up for new changes is to commit to doing something for just thirty days. You can even tell yourself that after those thirty days are up, you are free to quit if you so choose. People often fear or loathe change, so committing to something for just thirty days makes it seem a bit more manageable.

You may also want to use triggers to help you form good habits. Triggers are little rituals people perform before engaging in an activity. You can use a healthy breakfast as a trigger to exercise, taking a short rest as a trigger to go to the gym, or watching your favorite TV show as a trigger to write in your journal.

Be realistic about the changes you want to make. If you really hate going to the gym, you're not going to show up on day thirty-one. Instead, buy some exercise tapes and use your living room as your workout room. Buy an exercise bike or take long walks around your neighborhood. Try to incorporate some fun into the changes you want to make. The changes should create more joy than pain in your life.

CHAPTER 13

Practicing Wellness

WELLNESS IS THE process of consciously committing to growth and improvement in all areas of your life, whether it's your health, your career, your relationship, or your mental well-being. It requires that you take responsibility for the quality of your life. From here on in, it's essential that you create your own prescription for living, one that incorporates good habits for physical and emotional health. Being the best you can be will help you face any challenges MS throws your way. Wellness asks that you pay attention to every part of you and not just the MS.

Physical Wellness

Here's a news flash: Even though you have MS, you're still susceptible to colds, toothaches, and rainy days. It's easy to think that now that you've been unwittingly handed a chronic illness, you've filled your quota for physical maladies. Not true. You'll still need to go to the dentist and have regular checkups with your doctor. Paying careful attention to your overall health will make you stronger and better able to cope with the days ahead.

Your body is a highly complex mechanism capable of performing millions of functions on its own. Even so, it needs a little help from you to keep functioning properly. The decisions you make every day—such as drinking water rather than soda, or exercising instead of watching TV—may seem small. But taken together, day after day, year after year, they have a big impact on your life. The trick to healthy living is making small changes at first—changes in diet, exercise, and lifestyle.

Fact

Smokers are more than twice as likely to develop MS, as compared to people who have never smoked, according to a study published in *Neurology*, a medical journal. The risk was increased for people whether they were smokers at the time they developed MS or were past smokers. The results of the study may provide clues about what causes MS.

Your neurologist isn't the best person to enlist to take care of your overall health. You'll want to schedule regular checkups with your family physician along with routine tests. Keep in mind that different tests are recommended for different age groups, so be sure to ask your primary care physician what tests he recommends for you. The NMSS has a brochure called Preventative Care Recommendations for Adults with MS. Call 1-800-FIGHT-MS to have one sent to you.

Nutrition

Despite a lot of anecdotal evidence, there are no diets that have been definitively shown to alter the course of MS. But it's no secret that good nutrition is vital to your well-being, and like everyone else, you need to pay attention to what you're putting into your body. Experts say most people think they're eating a lot better than they actually are.

While eating well may not cure MS, it does provide other benefits. Eating well can make you feel better physically. It's also another way in which you're taking control of your life.

The U.S. Department of Health and Human Services publishes dietary guidelines every five years to provide advice on good dietary habits. (Keep in mind that it's important to figure out what your own personal caloric needs are before changing your diet.)

Consume a variety of nutrient-dense foods and beverages within the basic food groups while choosing foods that limit the intake of saturated and trans fats, cholesterol, added sugars, salt, and alcohol.

You should meet the recommended intakes by adopting a balanced eating pattern. (Check out *www.mypyramid.gov* for hints and clickable tools to aid you in your choices.)

 Alert

> Medications (such as corticosteroids) and inactivity can increase the risk for osteoporosis. Talk to your doctor about taking calcium supplements if you are currently taking these medications.

While that advice may seem pretty straightforward, most people get a little confused when it comes to good nutrition. In a nutshell, you'll want to get your nutrition from a variety of food groups, mainly grains, fruits, vegetables, lean meats, and low-fat dairy products. Increase your consumption of complex carbohydrates such as legumes, whole grains, and starchy vegetables. And while taking a multivitamin every day may be a good idea, vitamin and mineral supplements are not a substitute for a balanced and nutritious diet. Eat five servings of fruits and vegetables per day. One cup of sliced apple constitutes a serving, so it doesn't take much to incorporate it into your daily meal plan. To get a healthy variety of foods, think color. Eating fruits and vegetables of different colors gives your body a wide range of valuable nutrients, such as antioxidants, fiber, folate, and potassium. Green spinach, orange sweet potatoes, black beans, yellow corn, purple plums, and red watermelon are good examples.

Try to serve fish at least twice a week as a main course. It's rich in essential fatty acids and provides numerous health benefits, especially for the heart. And whenever possible, eat whole, fresh, and unprocessed foods. Even when you eat them in smaller amounts, you're likely to get a well-rounded group of nutrients.

Question

Does sunscreen have an effect on vitamin D?
Sunscreen inhibits the conversion of vitamin D to its active form, and since there is some evidence that some people with MS are deficient in this vitamin, it's a good idea to rely on dietary sources to meet your daily requirements. You might also consider putting sunscreen on fifteen minutes after you've been out in the sun.

Although it can be hard, make smart food choices wherever you are—the grocery store, work, or at a restaurant—by planning ahead. Pack a nutritious lunch before leaving for work, have a weekly menu planned before you go shopping, and ask for steamed or broiled dishes when dining out. You'll want to vary your protein choices with more beans, nuts, peas, and seeds.

It's no secret that most people could stand to trim the fat from their diets. Use vegetable oil instead of butter, choose fat-free or low-fat dairy products, and trim the skin from poultry. Replace red meat with chicken, poultry, or fish. It's also smart to see sweets as an occasional treat instead of a food group. (Yep, that's a tough one!)

Be resourceful! Eating well doesn't have to be boring.

Incorporating MS into Your Diet

According to the NMSS, people with MS have a few special dietary considerations, which makes sense since medications and inactivity can have an impact on your health. Here are some points to consider:

- If you're less active than you used to be, you may want to decrease your caloric intake.
- If you're underweight, you'll want to pinpoint the cause. Lack of appetite and fatigue can cause weight loss, which in turn can undermine your health.
- If urinary tract infections and other bladder problems are an issue for you, increase your fluid intake. Not getting enough fluids can increase fatigue and constipation. Water is always your best bet, but low-calorie sodas will also suffice in moderation.
- If constipation is a problem (and it's common in MS), an increase in fiber can be your greatest ally. Certain medications make constipation worse, as does dehydration and inactivity. Twenty-five grams of fiber a day is a good goal. Whole-grain breads, brown rice, and dried beans are a few sources of fiber that are helpful.

Exercise

It wasn't long ago that people diagnosed with MS were told to go home, relax, and conserve their energy, but we now know that advice doesn't rate very high on the wisdom scale. The old adage "If you don't use it, you'll lose it," has some truth. Inactivity and lack of exercise leads to deconditioned muscles that may worsen fatigue, weakness, and walking problems—and, ultimately, your quality of life. Part of your strategy, then, to achieve a state of well-being, is to find some form of exercise that fits well with your lifestyle and your own particular needs.

Exercising on a daily basis helps your body become more efficient at burning calories, which may give you more energy throughout the day. Regular exercise also strengthens the immune system and reduces stress levels. It's also a great mood booster.

If that's not enough, be aware that exercise benefits your cardiovascular system and helps to build and maintain healthy bones, muscles, and joints while regulating appetite, bowel movements, and sleep patterns.

Essential

Your doctor can help you optimize your use of spasticity medications and exercise. It's usually very helpful to consult a physical therapist (PT) or occupational therapist (OT) to help you to construct an exercise routine that suits your needs.

Sizing Up Your Options

Perhaps you weren't keen on exercise before you had MS, or maybe you were jogging five miles every day and an altered form of exercise, such as yoga, doesn't excite you very much. Or maybe you're dealing with fatigue and exercise is the furthest thing from your mind. Hopefully you can coax yourself into thinking differently about exercise. Once you start reaping the benefits, you may not need much more convincing.

Before you reach for your sneakers, it's important to note that you may have to take certain precautions if you want your exercise campaign to be successful. Check with your doctor before jumping on the treadmill or heading to the gym. You want to be careful not to overdo it, as you can overwork your muscles and tire yourself out. It's also important to choose a workout that is appropriate for your level of ability. Your physical and occupational therapists can also assist you in selecting the best exercise program for you to follow. Following are some good options to consider when you're ready to get moving.

Stretching

Folks who experience spasticity or increased muscle tone can really benefit from simple stretching techniques. Stretching has been credited with decreasing muscle tightness and pain caused by muscle spasms. (Check out the NMSS brochure, *Stretching with a Helper for People with MS*, by visiting *www.nationalmssociety.org/download .aspx?id=332*, or by calling 1-800-FIGHT-MS.) Stretching can also help your posture and improve mobility. The nice thing about stretching is that, typically, you don't need any equipment.

The nice thing about stretching is that if one way of stretching isn't working for you, there are other ways you can stretch the same muscle or muscle group.

Question

Do MS symptoms worsen before or after the menstrual cycle?
Although further study is needed, some women report that their symptoms worsen prior to their periods. Some small studies have shown that some women experience worsening of their chronic symptoms during this premenstrual period.

Strength Training

No, it's not just for bodybuilders anymore. Strength training is good for everyone, as it reduces body fat, increases lean muscle mass, strengthens your bones, and burns calories. Muscle mass diminishes naturally with age; combined with inactivity, this can lead to weakness. Folks with MS benefit from weight training because it increases their capacity to perform daily tasks and decreases the chance of injury. Increased endurance and strength are also benefits. A PT or OT can help you assess your current muscle strength and design a program that works for you.

Yoga

This form of exercise combines breathing techniques with a series of poses that are held to increase strength, flexibility, and balance. Yoga has proven to be a good activity for people with MS, as it can be adapted to an individual's ability. Studies have shown that yoga can lessen fatigue in people with MS as well as increase energy levels. Some chapters of the NMSS offer yoga classes. Call 1-800-FIGHT-MS for more information.

Water Exercise

Swimming or aerobic exercise in cool water is enthusiastically embraced by people with MS who have added it to their exercise regimen. Physical activity that is difficult on dry land is often easier in the water, and there are folks with disabilities who say that in water, they can move in ways they thought were no longer possible. It's a great way to keep joints and muscles active and to burn calories. An added bonus is that the water cools down the body's core temperature—something people with MS can appreciate. Look for aquatic programs in your area. Your local NMSS may have a list of them.

Aerobic Exercise

Studies show that aerobic exercise can effectively reduce fatigue in people with MS. The goal of aerobics is to get the blood pumping through the heart and increase your pulse and respiration. There are all sorts of ways you can increase your heart rate without joining a gym or an exercise class. Taking a brisk walk, swimming, and using a treadmill are good ways to get aerobic exercise.

Just Do It

If you've ever made a New Year's resolution, you know what can happen to good intentions. Exercise is one of those things that can be hard to stick with. The trick is to find creative ways to get over the hurdles that are preventing you from creating a healthy lifestyle. If fatigue is standing in your way, try to commit to just five minutes of exercise a day. Then work your way up slowly to ten minutes in a span of time that is comfortable for you.

Getting exercise doesn't have to be a big production. There are plenty of ways for everyone to get moving—including those with mobility issues—without breaking the bank or altering your schedule too much. The idea is to get your body moving and your heart pumping. Here are some good ways to get your heart beating faster without a lot of fuss:

- Do chair exercises. Seated aerobic exercises are designed to increase your heart rate from a sitting position. Seated jumping jacks, heel-toe exercises, and foot bounces are good exercises to start with. Go online for ideas or try YouTube for visual instruction. Try to do fifteen minutes a day at first and work your way up to thirty minutes if you can. You can also break it up into several segments per day.
- Take the stairs instead of the elevator.
- Don't take the closest parking spot, however happy you are to have found it.
- At work, use the restroom on another floor.
- Get an exercise video. Exercise videos allow you to get moving in the safety and comfort of your own home. Check out fitness shows on your cable channels as well.
- Walk with a pet for additional motivation to exercise.
- See cleaning the house as an opportunity to exercise. Use good posture when doing the dishes, tighten your abdominals when bending, and really put some muscle into vacuuming.

You want to make your exercise routine a vital and fulfilling part of your journey to wellness, so it's important to take safety into consideration to avoid injury, exhaustion, or discomfort. Start off moderately. Make fitness a part of your routine but don't push yourself too hard. Get used to one level of activity before increasing the length or intensity. It's always a good idea to warm up first, starting out gently and then slowly increasing respiration and circulation.

Remember to cool down after exercising; it helps the body to recover from the workout. And don't forget to hydrate: The body needs four to eight ounces of water every twenty minutes to replace water loss when exercising. Also, set realistic goals and reward yourself when you've reached them.

Fact

Studies show that it's not money or material possessions that make people happy but spending time with others. Happy people also pursue personal growth and intimacy and don't judge themselves by other people's yardsticks. A 2005 study also showed that people with illnesses or disabilities can be just as happy as those without medical conditions, indicating that people have the ability to adapt to new circumstances.

Emotional Well-Being

Happiness is really the holy grail of life, and whether you realize it or not, almost everything you do is aimed at making yourself happy. The desire to be happy ranks at the top of most everyone's list; studies show that people put it ahead of health, status, and fame. Research has revealed that people who are happy live longer, are healthier, and have better relationships. Americans in particular place tremendous value on pursuing it.

Statistics show that less than 30 percent of people report being truly happy; 25 percent of Americans claim they are depressed. Some research conducted on twins suggests that our happiness levels may be genetically influenced, but that doesn't mean our happiness levels are fixed. There's a lot people can do to be happier in life.

First, it's important to define what makes you happy as a human being. Studies show that good relationships, meaningful work, community ties, and personal freedom all contribute to our happiness quotient.

Cultivating Happiness

Having MS or another chronic illness does not preclude you from happiness. People have the remarkable ability to adapt to changes in their lives, including illness, disability, change in employment status, or the death of a family member. It's important to remember, though, that happiness isn't something you stumble upon. It's something that you work on and cultivate. It's less a place you reach than it is the process of getting there.

How can you find ways to be happier? Here are some suggestions researched by Dr. Mihaly Csikszentmihalyi, who has done extensive study on happiness:

1. **Realize that enduring happiness doesn't come from success.** People adapt to changing circumstances whether the circumstance is wealth or a physical disability.
2. **Take control of your time.** Happy people feel in control of their lives. One can master her use of time by setting goals and breaking them into daily objectives. Though people often overestimate how much they can accomplish in a day, you generally underestimate how much you can accomplish if you work on it bit by bit.
3. **Act happy.** Sometimes you can act yourself into a frame of mind. Just by smiling, one can begin to feel better; just as scowling can result in feeling negative. So, put on a happy face and see if you can trigger the happiness emotion.
4. **Seek work and leisure that engage your skills.** Happy people are often in a zone called "flow"—an absorption in a task that challenges them without overwhelming them.
5. **Join the "movement" movement.** A large amount of research has revealed that aerobic exercise, as well as yoga and meditation, not only promotes health and energy, it also helps to alleviate mild depression and anxiety.

6. **Give your body the sleep it wants.** Happy people tend to live active, vigorous lives, yet reserve time for rejuvenating sleep and solitude. Sleep deprivation can result in fatigue, diminished alertness, and gloomy moods.

7. **Give priority to close relationships.** Close, intimate friendships with those who care deeply about you can help you get through difficult times. Resolve to nurture your closest relationships by not taking them for granted, show kindness to them, affirm them, and share time together.

8. **Focus beyond the self.** It is important to reach out to those in need. While happiness can increase helpfulness, doing good also makes one feel good.

9. **Keep a gratitude journal.** Taking time each day to pause and to reflect on some positive aspect of your life (such as friends, family, health, freedom, education, natural surroundings) may increase your well-being.

10. **Nurture your spiritual self.** For many, focus on spirituality and religion provides a support community, a way to look beyond self, and a sense of purpose and hope. Research indicates that people who nurture religious or spiritual interests tend to be happier and cope better with crises.

All of these suggestions can be adapted to your own needs and limitations. If fatigue has kept you from cultivating relationships with friends, try to find a proactive way to address the issue. Can you plan a weekly or monthly get-together at your house? Suggest a potluck dinner so everyone shares a portion of the prep work. Speak with your neurologist about ways in which you can improve your sleep habits or ask him to help you establish an exercise routine. If you're feeling housebound, volunteer at your local chapter of the NMSS or hospital for a few hours a week. The point is to decide what makes you happy, then assess areas of your life where you may be deficient and set out to improve the situation. You, and you alone, must take responsibility for your own happiness.

Living Well with MS

One of the unexpected consequences of living with MS is that you may discover how to live a more balanced life than someone who does not have your diagnosis. And while that may not seem like much of a bonus prize, it has some important implications.

You've probably had to take a step back from work, carpooling, entertaining, and the other demands of your busy schedule on more than one occasion to focus on yourself and some aspect of MS, whether it was a doctor's appointment, medical testing, or simply getting some rest. Searching for ways to comfort yourself after the impact of your diagnosis or learning how to calm your own fears regarding the future are examples of ways that you've been using your condition as a catalyst for growth. Emotional well-being may require that you find some greater meaning in your journey with MS, whether it's learning more about yourself, creating a spiritual foundation, or striving to take better care of your health. Whether you realize it or not, you are already on that road; you can't endeavor to do anything in life without somehow unveiling a little bit more of who you are.

Essential

"Chronic illness doesn't come with an instruction manual," says author Susan Milstrey Wells in her book *A Delicate Balance: Living Successfully with Chronic Illness*. Wells gives advice on finding a doctor, accepting illness, working with a chronic disease, maintaining relationships, and searching for both conventional and unconventional treatments.

Being well or overcoming an illness doesn't necessarily mean being cured. It means caring for your MS while gradually trying to make your life happier and more fulfilling. It means achieving a level of well-being despite MS. Even though you may be adding new MS symptoms to your life along the way, you can also add new abilities and strengths.

Achieving a state of well-being is not an easy task. So many well-meaning books and people advise you to "take control of your life," while glossing over the difficulties involved in doing so. Learning to balance MS with the rest of your life is a tall order and it's not going to happen overnight; after all, life wasn't easy before you had MS. It helps to remember, though, that there is a zone—a state of mind— that is accessible to you, even during your worst days. It's a place where illness cannot enter, where happiness is a state of mind and not a stroke of luck. It's also a place where your life has a sense of purpose and meaning.

Barriers to Self Care

There are all kinds of reasons folks don't exercise, eat right, or take control of their emotional health. Most people cite time and resistance to change as the biggest barriers, but the truth is, a lot of it comes down to a lack of motivation. People often need a reason to change; in truth they need to redefine their reasons for living. For example, someone who is lonely may not feel motivated to employ self-care measures. He may feel depressed and unsupported by family or community. "What's the point?" he wonders. Low self-esteem and putting others before our own needs are also barriers to self-care. Here are a few more to consider:

- **Lack of support.** In this highly mobile society, too many people are left stranded and isolated. Not everyone has access to friends and family, and not everyone knows how to ask for help. Reaching out to neighbors, community services, and support groups are a few of the ways to find support. Several words sum it up in a nutshell: find, request, and accept support.
- **Lack of hope.** Hopelessness arrives at your door in a myriad of ways. Your economic situation can muddle your life, along with isolation and lack of self-confidence. There are a lot of ways to build self-efficacy; you must look for the resources,

information, and inspiration to find hope. Seeing a social worker or a psychotherapist may be a good place to start.

- **Resistance to change.** One of the biggest barriers to achieving a state of wellness is the resistance to change. You may have good reasons for cherishing bad habits, but there's also a certain amount of discomfort that goes along with changing your life. People are creatures of comfort and often resist creating new habits and routines.

Physical and emotional well-being are the cornerstones to living a full and happy life. Your goal is to be the best you can be, even with your concerns, health problems, and daily struggles. Find a new yardstick to measure your growth and success. Realize that certain aspects of your life have changed, and that you may have to redefine your goals. The point is to keep reaching beyond what you perceive as your limits and strive for more. Exercising just five minutes a day is a goal; so is looking for new relationships or starting new hobbies. Whatever your limits, you can always feel better, more hopeful and more alive.

CHAPTER 14

Mind and Body

IT'S TRUE THAT you cannot control everything that happens to you. All humans have experienced the feeling of powerlessness as certain events unfolded in their lives. As a person who has been diagnosed with MS, you are likely not a stranger to that feeling. What is essential to understand, however, is that although you can't always control what happens to you, you can control the way in which you live and how your body handles the stressors that you face. In the past several decades science has been studying this notion—that the mind and the body are intricately connected.

Mind-Body Connection

Your body responds to the way you think, feel, and act. When you are experiencing poor emotional health, you may not be taking care of yourself as best as you can by exercising, eating right, or following your doctor's orders. A good goal for anyone, then, is to try to achieve the highest sense of well-being that is possible. You want to live the happiest and healthiest life within the context of MS.

Mind-body medicine integrates modern scientific medicine, psychology, nutrition, exercise, physiology, and belief to enhance the natural healing capacities of body and mind. Many practitioners use a three-pronged approach when it comes to illness: conventional drugs, surgery (if needed), and self-care, which includes mind-body interventions.

There are many ways you can achieve a state of well-being, and although some may seem somewhat foreign to you, they may be worth investigating. You want to have a toolbox full of coping strategies so you are better equipped to handle the challenges of living with MS.

Fact

You've heard the warnings that stress can lead to heart disease, or that inadequate rest can leave you more vulnerable to colds and flu. Research has also shown that people who get their feelings out in the open, who have the support of community and friends, and who are able to distract themselves from pain, are typically more happy and hopeful and also better able to cope with an illness.

Spirituality

Some people erroneously think that spirituality and religion are one and the same. Religion is defined as a set of beliefs generally held by a group of people defined by ritual, prayer, and religious law. For the purposes of this chapter, spirituality is defined as an individual's sense of peace, purpose, and connection to others, as well as one's beliefs about the meaning of life. Spirituality can be expressed in an organized religion or in other ways. In fact, many people consider themselves to be both spiritual and religious. Some people find spirituality in religion, others through music, art, or an appreciation of nature.

Some research suggests that having a sense of spirituality may make an individual with an illness feel better. Spiritual and religious well-being may be associated with improved quality of life by reducing anxiety and depression, reducing a sense of isolation, and bestowing others with a feeling of personal growth, despite having an illness.

Some believe that the mind, body, and spirit are all inextricably linked in a complex mosaic that affects our health and well-being, although it's not crucial to believe that in order to develop a spiritual life. Spirituality can also be seen as a way to feel more content and at peace with your life. Developing a spiritual perspective means being willing to entertain the concept that you are more than just a physical being, but have complex emotional, social, and spiritual needs that factor into your health.

Essential

> Spirituality is unique to each individual, but spirit most often refers to the deepest part of you, that part that brings meaning to your world. It gives you a sense of who you are and what your purpose is. It is the part of you that allows you to cultivate strength and hope.

How then, do you improve your spiritual health? First, it might help you to assess your own spiritual health. Do you feel a sense of worth, hope, commitment, and peace? Do you have a positive outlook? If you feel despair, or entertain feelings of emptiness and conflict, these may be signs of spiritual unrest. Here are seven ways you can improve your spiritual health:

1. **Take time for yourself each day.** The amount of time isn't crucial. Walking or just sitting for fifteen minutes daily may be refreshing and energizing. You may want to include spiritual practices in your free time, such as meditation, praying, or yoga. The point is, spending time alone and away from persistent task-oriented activity gives you time to focus on your own spiritual well-being.

2. **Manage your time.** In this day and age, very little time is spent on personal interests. Learning to manage your time wisely allows you to lessen your anxiety and factor in some quality moments for yourself.

3. **"Hug a tree."** Spending time in nature promotes feelings of solitude and peace. Eat your lunch on a patch of grass. Read a book in the shade. Or lie on a hammock and feel the breeze across your face. Having fresh flowers on your table is another way to let a little of the outside in. Brief interactions with nature can restore a sense of peace in an otherwise hectic world.

4. **Recognize the endless possibilities.** There is an endless amount to learn in this world. Buy a telescope and gaze at the stars. Learn to speak French. Study philosophy. Have you ever made a "Life List"? A Life List expresses all of the things you've always wanted to do. If you can't visit Spain right now, you can travel there on the Internet. You can learn to make paella. You can throw a party with sombreros and piñatas. The point is to engage your mind. No one should stop learning after graduating from high school or college.

5. **Find meaning in the small things.** In a world where bigger is best, we often overlook the simple grace and meaning in the small things. There's something to be said for a quiet afternoon reading the paper or making a cake from scratch. Many people with illnesses have reported a renewed sense of appreciation for things they once overlooked—something as simple as a sunset or the smell of a fire burning on a cold winter day.

6. **Find a psychotherapist.** A good therapist can help you strategize for the future and help you to identify roadblocks to your happiness. Also, learning to vent or share your feelings in a healthy way is imperative to your emotional well-being.

7. **Set goals.** Since you cannot change the fact that you have MS, it is important to identify the things you can change. What would make you happier in your life? How do you attain those

things? Setting goals is imperative to your well-being, as long as you don't become too task orientated. When you identify some manageable goals you start to challenge yourself. You use your mind and creative energy to put your life in motion.

Changing your behaviors can improve your spiritual health. Seeking connections with others by joining a support group or volunteering can help you to feel more a part of your communities and thus less isolated. Practicing self-love and self-care is important, whether it be developing new hobbies, committing to an exercise routine, or spending time alone. It is important to always try to feel a greater sense of yourself.

Mind-Body Techniques

Mind-body medicine is an approach to healing that uses the power of thoughts and emotions to positively influence our well-being. Its goal is to activate the relaxation response and reduce the stress response. The techniques exert their influence on the hypothalamus, the switching station in the brain, which exercises control over the autonomic nervous system (which controls heart rate, and blood pressure), the endocrine system (glandular), and the immune system. Many hospitals are implementing mind-body clinics to reduce pain and stress and facilitate the well-being of their patients.

Meditation

Meditation, one of the most common mind-body interventions, is a conscious mental process that induces what is called the relaxation response. MRI has been used to identify the brain regions that are active during meditation. This research suggests that various parts of the brain known to be involved in attention and in the control of the autonomic nervous system are activated by meditation, indicating that meditation has an effect on our physiology. A more recent study showed that meditation produces significant increases in left-sided brain activity, which is associated with positive emotional states. There is also suggestive evidence that meditation may improve immune function, improve sleep, and reduce depression.

Fact

Meditation is the practice of quieting the mind. To practice meditation, you concentrate on a single sound, a word, an image, or your breath, striving to empty your mind of thoughts and increase the awareness of self. The National Institute of Health has an informative brochure on meditation. Visit *http://nccam.nih.gov/health/meditation/meditation.pdf* for more information.

Some types of meditation involve movement, such as yoga, while others require that you sit perfectly still. Some people even consider prayer to be a form of meditation. There are plenty of books and tapes on the market that can teach you meditation, or you may want to take a class with other beginners.

Relaxation Techniques

Along with meditation, there are two other relaxation techniques in mind-body medicine:

1. **Autogenic training.** This technique uses visual imagery and body awareness to put a person into a deep state of relaxation.
2. **Progressive muscle relaxation.** This technique involves slowly tensing and then releasing muscle groups in the body, starting in the toes and finishing with the muscles in the head.

It may be useful to try various techniques at least once and then find the combination that works best for you. Ideally, you should do the exercises daily. Relaxation techniques are designed to train your mind to become less responsive to stress. They may help you to maintain the calm and peaceful feelings you obtain throughout the day.

Guided Imagery

Guided imagery is a form of meditation in which you direct your thoughts and imagination toward a relaxed and focused state. There are different ways to approach this practice, including the use of tapes, an instructor, or scripts, but the purpose here is to use creative imagery to induce a state of relaxation. Some people imagine beautiful encounters with nature, while others may envision a particularly wonderful day they have had.

Most people are aware that negative thoughts often provoke unhealthy reactions. Thinking of someone who makes you nervous, such as your boss or your mother-in-law, may cause you to feel butterflies in your stomach. That's the premise of guided imagery—-the belief that positive and peaceful thoughts will promote well-being in your body.

Question

How does guided imagery work?
When using a human guide or a tape for guided imagery, you are often guided toward a relaxed state where you imagine all the details of a safe, comfortable place, such as a beach or a garden. This relaxed state may aid in healing, learning, creativity, and performance. It may help you feel more in control of your emotions and thought processes, which may improve your attitudes, health, and sense of well-being.

Hypnosis

Hypnosis can be a helpful therapy in MS. It may encourage relaxation, control anxiety and pain, and boost mood and optimism. Hypnosis is a state of consciousness resembling sleep, an altered, relaxed state of mind, where people are often open to suggestion.

Self-hypnosis is another way we can induce this state of relaxation, although the hypnotic state will not be as deep as when you are hypnotized by someone else. Self-hypnosis can be used to reduce feelings of anxiety and promote relaxation. There are plenty of books and Internet resources to teach you more about hypnosis.

 Alert

While people often associate hypnosis with entertainment, it's used as a clinical tool, especially in psychotherapy where people are trying to change behaviors, such as kicking a smoking habit or losing weight. It's important to find a trained health provider, such as a clinical psychologist, for this therapy.

Biofeedback

Biofeedback is another type of unconventional therapy that uses the mind to control the body. Using feedback from various monitoring procedures and equipment, a biofeedback specialist can teach you to control certain involuntary body responses, such as brain activity, blood pressure, heart rate, and muscle tension.

Fact

Biofeedback may be helpful in treating many medical conditions and symptoms, including headaches, incontinence, high blood pressure, and epilepsy. Clinical trials are evaluating biofeedback in other conditions as well. You can receive biofeedback training in hospitals, physical therapy offices, and medical centers. Ask your specialist to recommend a biofeedback program.

During a biofeedback session, a specialist will place electrical sensors on various parts of your body that will measure your physiological response to stress. The goal is to help the patient gain some voluntary control over autonomic body functions. For example, say you are having tension headaches. Biofeedback may show you that you are tensing certain muscles that are causing the headaches. In essence, biofeedback teaches you to become aware of—and control—involuntary functions that have a negative effect on your body.

Yoga

A study published in the journal *Neurology* found that yoga improved fatigue in people with MS. Several other studies on cancer patients showed that those who practiced yoga slept better and required less sleep medication. Some of the reported benefits of yoga in people with MS include increased body awareness, release of muscular tension, increased coordination and balance, less fatigue, and better management of stress.

Prayer

Prayer is the most commonly used type of CAM; it's reported that nearly half of all Americans use some form of prayer in their lives. Researchers have recently begun to conduct studies on prayer to better understand if, and how, it may produce beneficial effects.

Researchers at the National Center for Complementary and Alternative Medicine (NCCAM) have seen some evidence that religious affiliation and religious practices are associated with health and mortality. What that means is that people with a spiritual connection may have a longer and healthier life. It may be that those who practice a religion have an effective way to cope with stress.

Prayer is an attempt to communicate with whatever you quantify as being greater than yourself, such as a deity, spirit, energy, or perhaps something you don't even label or identify. You may also look at prayer as a metaphor for hope. Typically, people pray for a positive outcome, such as good health or relief from a difficult situation. Prayer has a physiological effect on the body as it slows heart rate, lowers blood pressure, reduces stress and anxiety, and creates a sense of well-being. It can be done alone or in groups—in church with a prayer group.

Cognitive Behavior Therapy (CBT)

Much is said about how our thoughts influence our lives. This idea makes sense at a basic level, since much of what you do—from getting a drink of water to applying for a new job—originates as a thought.

Further, many of your thoughts are habitual, based on how you perceived something in the past. Perhaps you were once chased by a dog and now, even twenty years later, whenever you see a dog you react with fear and the fight-or-flight reaction. Your responses to dogs are still rooted in your thoughts about dogs, thoughts that were formed many years in the past. Cognitive behavior therapy strives to alter those thoughts and create a new response to stimuli, with the goal of relieving stress and anxiety.

CBT is based on the idea that your thoughts cause your feelings and behaviors, and that rather than try to change an impossible situation, you can change your thoughts about it to feel better. A good way to practice CBT is to find a therapist that specializes in it.

Do Mind-Body Techniques Work?

There is extensive evidence that stress suppresses the body's immune system. Researchers are currently using animal models to evaluate how psychological stress impacts the disease process, but it's already known that chronic stress can have a negative impact on the body's functioning, and in turn, have negative health implications. It stands to reason, then, that interventions to decrease stress may have health benefits.

Research is also recognizing that there are individual differences as to how quickly a wound heals. Stress and negative mood may be associated with slow wound healing.

Multiple studies of cancer patients suggest that mind-body interventions may improve mood, quality of life, and coping.

Perhaps the most encouraging aspect of mind-body medicine is that there is very little physical or psychological risk involved and the techniques are easy to learn.

Essential

Future research that focuses on mind-body medicine hopefully will yield new insights that may enhance the effectiveness of mind-body interventions. In the meantime, there is quite a bit of evidence that mind-body interventions have positive effects on psychological functioning and quality of life, and may be particularly helpful for people coping with chronic illness.

You may be interested in finding a mind-body program for people who live with chronic illness. Generally, its goal is to instill an understanding of how stress affects physical and emotional health, help patients reduce physical symptoms caused by stress, and teach patients to better cope with their illnesses. Call your local hospital to see if there is a mind-body program in your area.

CHAPTER 15

MS and Employment

WHEN IT COMES to employment and MS, it's important to keep your goals and aspirations in the forefront of your mind. Don't automatically assume that your symptoms will keep you from attaining all you want out of your career. No one knows what course your MS will take, and even if it catches you by surprise from time to time, you may find the world to be very accommodating. In this world of flextime and part-time, job sharing, and antidiscrimination laws, there are many options for those people with MS who are eager to keep a toehold in the working world.

To Tell or Not to Tell

Deciding whether or not to tell your employee that you have multiple sclerosis is a big decision. On the one hand, disclosure may garner you some much-needed support. On the other hand, you may confront some of the biases and misunderstandings that often surround MS and that could adversely (and unfairly) affect your career.

Common reasons that individuals with MS decide to disclose their illness to an employer include the following:

- Their symptoms are no longer invisible. They may be having problems with walking or muscle weakness and they can no longer hide their condition.
- Their symptoms are causing them to miss a lot of work and they're concerned about their job performance.
- They are interested in asking for accommodations at work that will allow them to perform better.

Since employers are increasingly exposed to chronic illness in the workplace, some have begun to offer flexible work schedules that address the needs of employees who have chronic conditions. In fact, one-third of U.S. companies offer options for increasing flexibility in work schedules.

Still, disclosure is a very personal issue and it's important to sit down and make a list of the pros and cons before making a decision. Be clear about your reasons for deciding to tell or not to tell. Consult a therapist, another professional, or a trusted friend to make sure your reasons are sound and logical and not based completely on emotions such as fear.

The Multiple Sclerosis International Federation (MSIF) has developed the Working Together Initiative to help educate and guide employers when it comes to dealing with MS-related issues in the workplace. They've also put together a list of advantages and disadvantages of telling your employer to help you make the right decision.

Advantages of Disclosure

Telling your employer of your diagnosis can bring peace of mind. Many people with MS report that "hiding is more stressful than telling." Disclosure also makes it easier, if the need arises, to discuss any workplace adaptations that might be necessary.

Being able to deal with people more honestly may also be an incentive to share your diagnosis. Having "cleared the air," you will have a better understanding of others' reactions to the fact that you have MS and of how you are likely to be perceived and treated by colleagues.

Sharing your diagnosis also releases you from the worry that a past employer or reference might inadvertently reveal the fact that you have a disability. And if a medical exam is required, your apprehension will be reduced knowing that the employer, insurance company, and other relevant parties are aware of your MS before the examination takes place.

Essential

An ongoing nationwide poll conducted by the NMSS found that 43 percent of adults who have had MS for twelve years or more retain employment. In some cases adjustments by you or your employer may have to be made, but flexibility and determination seem to be an important mix in maintaining a healthy and productive work life.

Disclosure also makes it easier to educate your colleagues regarding the true nature of the disease and allows you to discuss with your employer any future changes in your condition.

Fear of Disclosure

Fear of being discriminated against and missing out on opportunities such as a promotion or training venture often prevent people from disclosing their MS diagnosis. In fact, fear makes up most of the reasons why people are uncomfortable sharing this private matter in the workplace. People fear rejection from colleagues, or they fear losing their jobs—or not being offered a job at all.

Tips for Disclosure

If you do decide to share your diagnosis, approach the conversation with your boss (or whoever is appropriate, including a human resources manager) with as much professionalism as you do any work-related discussion. Talk specifics. Know what you'd like to get out of the conversation ahead of time, such as a more flexible schedule, a parking space closer to the door, or a work-from-home option. It's good to walk in with a solution in mind. Let your employer know you've considered the challenges and have planned strategies for working more effectively, making up for your absences, and accommodating other situations.

If you disclose your diagnosis (technically, you're not required to), be prepared to explain what MS is and how it affects you as an individual. Make sure to let your boss know that MS is variable by nature.

It's important to be familiar with discrimination laws before approaching someone at your company. Again, knowledge is power in this situation, and it's imperative to know your rights. It probably will not be necessary to recite them during your discussion, but you'll feel more confident knowing what the laws are and understanding what may constitute a reasonable request.

Essential

You might consider hiring a job coach (also called a career coach) to help guide you through the process of disclosure and to help you adjust to the workplace with a chronic illness. Look for a coach who has experience working with people who have chronic illnesses. Job coaches most often counsel by phone, so it's a convenient way to enlist some help. Visit *www.certifiedcareercoaches.com* for more information.

Americans with Disabilities Act (ADA)

The Americans with Disabilities Act was passed in 1990 and essentially prohibits discrimination based on disability. Private employers, state and local governments, employment agencies, and labor unions cannot discriminate against qualified individuals with disabilities in the application process, hiring, firing, promoting, salary, and other privileges of employment. In other words, if you have a disability, your rights are protected under the law. It's essential to understand exactly how the law applies to you in the workplace.

Fact

A recent study revealed that 125 million people in the U.S. work force have a chronic illness, which is defined as a medical problem that lasts a year or longer, limits what a person can do, and requires ongoing care. As people are living longer than ever before and thus working later into their lives, employers are confronted with the issues of chronic illness and disability in increasing numbers.

What Constitutes a Disability under the ADA?

This is an important question, because the law doesn't list certain diseases or conditions as a way to define disability. Instead, the ADA has a general definition of disability that each person must meet.

Under the ADA, a person is considered to have a disability if he has an impairment (usually a diagnosis), and the impairment substantially limits one or more major life activities (such as walking, seeing, hearing, reading, performing manual tasks, and so on). Additionally, an employee can meet the ADA's definition of disability by having a record (a medical record, for example) or being regarded as having a disability (by your doctor, perhaps, or even your boss).

This is where things can get a little sticky. It's up to the employer to determine whether or not you have a disability that requires some changes in the workplace. If your impairment is not known or is not obvious, your employer can ask for medical documentation to determine whether your disability substantially limits one or more life activities. Your employer may ask you to review the definition of disability provided by the ADA and determine for yourself whether you meet the criteria and then proceed with the accommodation request.

You may want (or you may be asked) to attach medical documentation to the request.

You are not required to divulge your diagnosis if you are not comfortable doing so. If pressed, you are entitled to be vague, saying only, for example, "I have a neurological condition." The law requires that you provide some verification from your physician that you have a disability, but doesn't specify that you divulge anything more. The letter from your doctor may only confirm that you have a "neurological condition" as well. Keep in mind that if the employer insists on knowing the diagnosis and the employee refuses to divulge it, the employer probably has a valid reason to refuse the request.

The easiest way around this, of course, is to divulge your diagnosis and have medical documentation from your physician at hand, but only you can decide what is comfortable for you based on your own set of unique circumstances regarding your health and your employment.

Question

Must I divulge my diagnosis to a prospective employer?
Employers may not ask job applicants about the existence, nature, or severity of a disability, although you may be asked about your ability to perform specific job functions. A job offer may be conditioned on the results of a medical examination, but only if the examination is required for all entering employees in similar jobs. Medical examinations of employees must be job related and consistent with the employer's business needs.

The ADA has muscle. In 2006, there were 15,575 formal charges of disability discrimination in the United States; 15,045 of the cases were resolved and $48.8 million in monetary benefits was recovered for the aggrieved parties. So, know that you have precedence—and the law—on your side if you have been treated unfairly at work.

Reasonable Accommodation

A reasonable accommodation is one that doesn't require your employer's undue hardship, meaning they should make every effort to meet your needs unless the accommodation is too expensive or disruptive for business. What is an undue hardship varies greatly given the size and financial resources of your company. A small company may not have the resources to accommodate. The ADA pertains to any employer who has fifteen or more employees, although individuals working for smaller companies may be entitled to similar protections under state and local laws. Keep in mind that an employer is not required to lower quality or production standards to accommodate a person with a disability, nor are they required to provide personal-use items such as glasses or hearing aids.

Unpaid leave is a reasonable form of accommodation, unless it will create a hardship for the employer. If you are reassigned to another position, it should be one that is of equal pay or equal status to the position you held before, or as close as possible. You must be qualified for the new position.

Fact

Under the ADA, reasonable accommodation includes making the facilities accessible for persons with disabilities. Employers are also required to restructure jobs, modify schedules, and reassign people to other positions if necessary. They must also modify or adapt the work environment and provide readers and interpreters when necessary.

Under the ADA, the responsibility falls on you to request accommodations, so you'll have to decide what you need and approach your employer yourself. Having a sound plan will help keep the conversation on track. If you'd like to explore adapting your work environment, know which assistive devices will work best for you. (Contact the Job Accommodation Network for ideas at *www.jan.wvu.edu*.) If you'd like to request a more flexible work schedule, have a specific plan in mind and be willing to listen to your employer's ideas. Hopefully, you can set the tone for teamwork and mutual cooperation.

The EEOC

The U.S. Equal Employment Opportunity Commission oversees enforcement of the employment title of the ADA. This is where you turn if you believe you are being discriminated against in the workplace, although your first line of defense is to make your best effort at working things out with your employer.

If you have been discriminated against, you are entitled to a remedy that will place you in the position you would have been in if the discrimination had never occurred, such as promotion, reinstatement, back pay, or reasonable accommodation, including reassignment. You may also be entitled to attorney's fees.

You can file a charge by contacting any EEOC field office, located in cities throughout the United States. To contact the EEOC, look in your telephone directory under "U.S. Government." For information and instructions on reaching your local office, call: 1-800-669-4000. Or look on the web at *www.eeoc.gov.*

Alert

A charge of discrimination generally must be filed within 180 days of the alleged discrimination (although you may have up to 300 days to file a charge if there is a state or local law that provides relief for discrimination on the basis of disability). However, to protect your rights, it is best to contact the EEOC promptly if discrimination is suspected.

Choosing Assistive Technology for the Workplace

Determining what assistive technology (AT) to request at the workplace can be challenging. You'll want to have a list of resources handy and employ useful decision-making strategies in order to find a successful fit. Consider this four-step process when choosing the right AT for the job:

1. Make a list of your symptoms and functional limitations. (A functional limitation involves difficulty in performing one or more specific activities, such as difficulty viewing the computer screen.) Think about how your symptoms might change over time. Be clear about what job tasks are difficult to perform.
2. Choose the AT. Make an informed decision based on the information gathered. Let your employer know what your selection or selections are. Be sure to explore whether there is technical assistance available and what sort of support the company offers to you and your employer.
3. Make sure you are properly trained and feel comfortable using the device once it arrives.
4. Monitor the device to make sure that you are using it properly, it is working as described, and it has fulfilled your expectations.

State vocational rehabilitation agencies are a great resource for information about assistive technology. They can evaluate and assess your situation and sometimes provide financial assistance to companies for accommodations. State Assistive Technology Act programs can provide technical assistance, consultation, product demonstrations, and equipment borrowing. For a list of state AT projects, and the number of the agency in your state, visit *www.jan.wvu.edu*. Utilize JAN's Searchable Online Accommodation Resource (SOAR). SOAR is an online tool that helps the user move through the accommodation process, suggests accommodation ideas, and provides resources, such as AT vendor contacts, for further exploration. To access SOAR, go to *www.jan.wvu.edu/soar/index.htm*.

Leaving Your Job

For most people, the decision to leave a job is a difficult one. Even if you've exhausted yourself trying to keep up with the demands of work and you're looking forward to a much-needed break, there are bound to be some emotions wrapped up in your decision to leave. Some people grapple with fears of "quitting" or giving up; others are more concerned with the financial aspects of their decision.

Beyond the emotional challenges, there are a myriad of details that will need your attention, including deciding when to make your exit, negotiating a severance package, and working on a financial plan. First and foremost, it's essential that you consult with members of your health care team so you can discuss your decision with them. They may have valuable input that will make you feel more comfortable about your decision.

Before making a decision, make sure to check your sick leave policy. You'll want to know how much, if any, has accumulated since you first started working at your place of employment.

The Family Medical Leave Act (FMLA) is an act that was passed in 1993 and provides unpaid, job-protected leave to eligible employees, both male and female, in order to care for their families or themselves for specified family and medical conditions.

Question

What are short-term disability plans?
Short-term disability plans allow you to leave work for a specified period of time. If your employer offers a plan, find out how much it pays. Short-term disability insurance covers a percentage of your lost salary should an injury or illness cause you to miss work for more than a few days. Payments generally kick in when you have exhausted any available sick leave.

FMLA provides eligible employees with up to twelve workweeks of unpaid leave in a twelve-month period for the birth, adoption, or foster-care placement of a child; care of a spouse, son, daughter, or parent with a serious health condition; or their own serious health condition that causes an inability to work. If you qualify and have unused FMLA leave time, your employer cannot deny you FMLA leave. You may wish to take advantage of the FMLA while you are making a decision about leaving work, or coordinate your exit in conjunction with the FMLA. Your employer must be covered by this law (i.e., be a company with fifty employees or more) and you must have worked for the employer for twelve months or more (and for at least 1,250 hours).

Long-term disability is also an option. Long-term disability insurance protects you from catastrophic illness or injury that permanently ends your ability to earn a paycheck. These policies usually pick up where short-term disability policies leave off. Some last only five or ten years, while others cover you until you are age sixty-five.

You may want to work with your doctor to set the date for your last day of work. Some HR professionals recommend not telling your employer more than two weeks before you leave, but this will depend on your own unique set of circumstances. Some people take advantage of their short-term disability and inform their employer that they won't be returning before the payments end.

Social Security Disability Insurance

Applying for SSDI can seem like a full-time job. There's a lengthy application process, a lot of paperwork to gather, and some teamwork required with your doctor. In short, you have to develop a strategy to pursue your claim effectively.

Most of the information shared here will focus on the application process as well as covering some old ground from past chapters. The SSDI requires you to prove the following:

- You are disabled under the SSDI's definition of disabled.

- You are entitled to benefits because you have worked a significant number of years and paid Social Security taxes.

While that may seem fairly straightforward, you must be able to prove that you are unable to do any kind of work on a full-time basis. Your doctor must also deem you "totally disabled." Any information you can add from another member of your health care team will also be helpful, such as a vocational rehabilitation counselor. Keep in mind, you will be granted SSDI not only because of your diagnosis, but because of your symptoms and limitations.

Alert

A diagnosis in itself does not prove disability. The quality of your medical records in describing your symptoms and limitations also plays a big factor, so you'll want to have the support of the physician (or physicians) who treat you. This is an important point. You have to make sure your medical providers and counselors support your claim. Without them, your chances of winning may be reduced.

One of the most confusing aspects of filing for SSDI is the plethora of forms that must be filled out. When doing so, now is not the time to overstate your abilities, putting the best slant on your illness. Rather, now is the time to be clear, concise, and honest about your symptoms and limitations. Also, consider yourself to be having a bad MS day when you fill out the paperwork; it's a more accurate assessment of what activity level you can sustain.

Another critical issue in your disability case is your symptoms—specifically the frequency, severity, and duration of your symptoms. You will want to briefly state your diagnosis, but then focus on your symptoms and how they limit not only your ability to work, but also your ability to function on a daily basis. Note any cognitive difficulties you are having and discuss the psychological effects of your condition, too. The Social Security Administration (SSA) recognizes four impairments in MS—gait, vision, cognitive problems, and fatigue—so you and your doctor will have to be able to document a major deficit in one these areas.

Essential

Nowadays, you can file your disability claim online. Or you can contact your nearest Social Security office to pick up an application or have one sent to you. (On the web, visit *www.ssa.gov.*) Once you've sent your application in and the Social Security Administration has reviewed your paperwork, you will be notified when and where an initial intake interview will take place, whether in the Social Security office or by phone.

During your initial interview with the SSA, you will go over your paperwork and sign several forms, including those that will allow the SSA to obtain your medical records.

Once the SSA has reviewed all of your information (application and medical records) they will make a decision known as an Initial Decision, sent as a written document. If you've been denied, your next step will be to file an appeal. This requires writing a Request for Reconsideration of your denial which must be submitted well within the sixty-day deadline. Because the SSA can deny your claim if you are even one day past this deadline, you should consider sending your request by certified mail. You may also submit additional medical information if you choose.

If a second denial notice is issued, you may put in a written request for a hearing, where you will appear in front of a judge. You may bring witnesses (friends, relatives, your doctor), although letters and other documentation will suffice. At this stage in the game, many people hire a lawyer who is skilled in disability law. The SSA maintains a list of lawyers' organizations that deal with these types of claims, as does the NMSS.

The last stop on the Social Security train is your local federal district court. The guidance of a skilled attorney would be prudent before, and if, you get to this point. Most work on a contingency basis, which means you would not render payment unless he is successful at getting you your benefits.

Fact

Because of the variable nature of MS, some people who have been receiving SSDI may decide they'd like to go back to work at some point. The SSA has a Ticket to Work program that offers various incentives to get you back into the work force if you so choose. Certain limitations and restrictions apply. For more information, visit the Social Security website at *www.ssa.gov/work*.

While deciding to leave the work force—even temporarily—can be a challenging decision, the good news is that there are plenty of options to consider. From long-term disability plans to the Family Medical Leave Act, there are an unprecedented number of programs designed to help you with the transition. The truth is that none of these things represents an easy solution. But doing what works best for you—and for your loved ones—should be your motivating factor. It may also help to know that should circumstances change, you always have the option of returning to work. Knowing that you can extend a measure of flexibility to the days ahead is reassuring.

CHAPTER 16

Family Life

LEARNING TO MANAGE and cope with MS is a family matter. MS may have an impact on your future plans, such as starting a family or taking a trip, and your current obligations, such as parenting or celebrating the holidays. In short, MS is likely to gather around the edges of your life, in big ways and small ways, and ask to come along for the ride. Finding room for it takes some patience and understanding. The trick is in learning to define your boundaries so that it doesn't take over your life.

Family Issues

Families have their own styles; some are open and communicative, while others tend to hold things inside. Your family's unique coping and communication styles will have a big impact on how it deals with the reality of MS. Mental health professionals stress the importance of cultivating new communication skills and strategies to keep the family functioning in a healthy way.

Living with MS involves more than the physical challenges created by the illness. It may also contribute to financial, relationship, and emotional challenges as well. Family life may be vastly altered if the primary wage earner is unable to work or if treatment requires long-term changes in the family routine and activities. Learning how to follow medical instructions, managing medication, working out financial challenges, and adapting to limitations and changes created by the illness all require learning new skills and ways of coping.

Essential

The Invisible Disabilities Advocate (IDA) is an organization devoted to people who live with invisible disabilities, which fits the criteria for many people living with MS. The IDA offers articles, booklets, pamphlets, links, an online support group, and a discount bookstore to help you and your loved ones forge the journey with limiting conditions. You can find them at *www.myida.org*.

Emotional Responses

Your diagnosis likely spurred a myriad of different responses in your family members. Here are some of the more common responses:

- **Depression.** It's common for family members to alternate between worrying about the person who was diagnosed and worrying about themselves. They may lose interest in activities or relationships or feel overwhelmed by new roles and responsibilities.
- **Anger.** Feeling angry at unexpected life events is normal. Family members may feel angry at a change in routine or family roles. Anger is often part of the acceptance process.
- **Guilt.** Family members can feel guilt over the misperception that they somehow caused the person to have MS. They may also feel guilty about the anger they are experiencing, or the feeling that they aren't doing enough to help.

221

- **Uncertainty.** Feeling concerned and unsure about the future is a common emotional response, particularly in young children. Life's new unpredictability can cause anxiety or depression.

Reaching out for support and help is important for families that are learning to cope with a life-altering event. Since we all cope in our own way, it's important to decipher what family members are experiencing, especially young children, who tend to lack effective communication skills. Seeking out support from mental health professionals may help ease anxiety and assist you in reworking your roles in the family system.

Question

How do I talk about the future with my kids?
You don't have to confront every "what if" but do explain some of your symptoms and what changes are likely to take place within the family. For example, you might say, "Some days, instead of going on a picnic, we might just stay home and play board games if it's too hot outside." As the parent, you're the best judge of what your child is capable of absorbing. Telling the truth from the start, though, will help to establish healthy communication down the road.

Talking to Your Kids

Honesty and openness are key when talking to children about your diagnosis. It's well known that kids are a lot more perceptive than we give them credit for. When they perceive changes in the house and in the family dynamics, they can become fearful if no explanation has been given. But it's also important to keep the discussion age- and child-appropriate.

When it comes to telling your children about your diagnosis, experts say the sooner the better. Be prepared to explain to them what MS is. Use illustrations or pamphlets to aid you.

During your conversation, children will usually respond with a few questions of their own. It's not uncommon to be asked whether or not you're going to die, to which, thankfully, you can respond that people with MS generally have a normal life expectancy. You may also want to reassure them that you are going to work hard to manage the disease by establishing a pattern of self-care. You might even consider involving your children in one or two of your routines, such as exercising with you or running to get the cotton balls before you give yourself an interferon injection.

Knowing what reactions are normal and abnormal in your child can help you figure out how they're coping with the news. Young children may develop their own physical maladies, such as stomachaches. They may want to cling a little tighter or sleep in your bed more than usual. Teenagers may choose to spend more time with their friends and less time at home. You'll want to be on the lookout for signs of depression or anxiety down the road—trouble at school, problems with friends, anything unusual that concerns you—but the important thing is to convey that there is nothing wrong with how they feel. Let them know it is okay to be angry or upset and give them a safe place to express it.

Before having a family meeting, you'll also want to get a handle on your own feelings. Experts say that once you have come to terms with your feelings, it's easier to help the children come to terms with theirs.

Community Resources

Your physician is a great resource in providing referrals for mental health counselors or community-based support. Here are some potential resources to consider when looking for support for family issues:

- Pediatric offices usually have connections to mental health professionals and can make appropriate referrals when counseling or psychotherapy is needed.

- There are some great books on coping with chronic illnesses. The NMSS also has some great brochures to help you cope with MS, including brochures for your children to read. Take a look online at *www.nationalmssociety.org/brochures* or call 1-800-FIGHT-MS.
- Children's museums and other museums often have exhibits or displays dealing with the human body and health. Educating your child about MS can be used as an opportunity to spend time together.
- Churches and synagogues often offer counseling or host support groups for children or families that are dealing with a chronic illness at home.

Children need support and understanding during this process. Since MS is a complex disease, it's not always easy to explain. Being educated about MS and being able to describe it well is important—and challenging. Experts say that given the right tools to help them cope, children can weather the changes in the family and emerge as healthy and well-adjusted kids. What happens to the parent impacts all family members, but when children are allowed to participate in the discussions and feel a part of the situation, it benefits everyone.

Changing Roles

After a family member is diagnosed with MS, family roles can shift over time. These changing roles in family, work, and social situations can create additional adjustment problems for everyone. Children may be called upon to help out more; husbands may have to add on additional household duties, or perhaps the main breadwinner has opted to scale down to part-time work. When roles change, you have to learn to redefine yourself and rethink your established duties or routines within the family system. How much the roles of family members change is largely dependent on how well the member with MS is doing, both physically and mentally.

Essential

When it comes to changing roles, we may still have a way to go. One study found that working mothers average eighteen hours per week of housework, plus ten to fifteen hours per week of child care, while fathers average three hours of housework and two hours of child care per week.

Along with roles come certain social and family expectations for how those roles should be fulfilled, so it's important to add flexibility into your own needs and expectations. Here are some tips to guide you in adapting to new roles within the family:

- **Establish clear roles.** Identify the roles played within your family system. Individual family members should clearly understand what is expected of them. It may be helpful to make a list for each family member to follow.
- **Allow for flexibility.** Being able to change roles is integral to a healthy family. Roles in all families can change over time, not just in families living with MS. Healthy families have the ability to adapt: The stay-at-home mother, for example, may head back to work, which might be a big adjustment for the rest of the family. Changing your expectations and adopting flexibility is an important strategy when coping with changes in the family structure.
- **Allocate roles fairly.** Roles should be spread among the various members so that no one is asked to take on too much responsibility. Problems can arise if one person is asked to take on too many roles. A full-time working mother cannot be expected to put in forty hours a week and then take on the lion's share of household duties. Everyone in the family should be expected to take on appropriate roles of responsibility.
- **Teach responsibility.** All family members should take their roles seriously and do their best to fulfill their duties. A healthy

family system is dependent on each person taking responsibility for himself. In families where clear, flexible roles exist, individual members will be much more likely to take their responsibilities seriously.

- **Family assessment.** It's a good idea to take stock of your family's strengths and weaknesses and take steps to improve the family system. Having good communication skills comes into play here. Schedule family meetings and take stock of how well things are going.

It is important for a family to maintain a good quality of life. Being able to give and receive love, enjoy pleasurable activities together, and sustain hope as a family unit are important characteristics of a healthy family.

Alert

The benefits of family dinners have been heralded for years by social scientists. A number of studies show that children who eat dinner with their families regularly are less likely to get involved with drugs and alcohol than those who do not. They also tend to get better grades, exhibit less stress, and eat better.

Communication Is the Key

Each family has its own unique coping style so it's no wonder there's not a "one size fits all" when it comes to communicating. Talking about changes or problems that arise in the family can be difficult. One person in the family may feel comfortable bringing up something "unpleasant," while another has been raised to live comfortably with the big elephant in the room that everyone has been tiptoeing around. Communication is so essential to a healthy family that it's really important to get help learning how to talk to one another about what's going on if it seems as if everyone is avoiding important issues. If one of your children feels anxious about your diagnosis and is not expressing it, it is bound to surface in other ways—some of which may be unhealthy, such as sleeping disturbances. If you feel overloaded with spring cleaning in the yard during a relapse, it's important to communicate your feelings in a way that will promote a solution rather than resentment. The guidelines to effective communication promote respect for all individuals and include being a good listener:

- **Don't be afraid to ask for help!** Rather than assuming other family members are certain of their tasks, point out what needs to be done.
- **Use "I" messages.** Rather than saying "You are not helping enough," use "I" statements, such as "I feel frustrated when I'm left to do all of the chores." These messages help others to feel less defensive when you're speaking to them. Your goal is to express your point of view.
- **Compromise.** Rather than trying to win an argument, you're looking for solutions. Healthy communication involves finding a resolution that both sides can be happy with.
- **Be clear.** MS can be deceiving. You may be standing there in your shirt and tie, looking as if you just had a great day at work, and all you really want to do is put your feet up and watch the news. Since so many MS symptoms are invisible, it's important to express your needs without assuming that others know how you're feeling.
- **Take a timeout.** Sometimes you might need to take a break from a topic and wait for clearer heads to prevail. But don't give up. If something needs to be discussed, revisit the issue again when you've had a few moments to collect yourself.
- **Find support.** If communication within your family has broken down or is difficult, seeing a family therapist can help. A therapist can help break the silence or resolve conflict and also teach coping skills. Avoiding conflict, being defensive, blaming others, and not actively listening are a few of the common communication barriers that need to be resolved.

Effective communication is an important characteristic of strong families and is one of the factors that helps them get through hard times. Even though communication patterns are learned over a long period of time, it's possible to build new communication skills.

Fact

Polls by the American Psychological Association have found that the leading factors preventing many people from seeking mental health treatment are financial reasons. Being unable to pay standard fees should not necessarily prevent someone who is having emotional or behavioral problems from getting quality treatment. Mental health clinics run by nonprofit agencies, universities, and state and local governments provide therapy services on sliding fee scales based on a person's income and ability to pay.

Keeping It Together

No matter what your role in the family has been thus far, it's likely that you're going to have to restructure your life in small or big ways to ensure that you're taking good care of yourself. This means that family roles may have to change, good communication skills must be learned, and flexibility will have to be exercised. Some people with MS find that they have to change very little in their households, while others may have more changes to contend with. Just as you created a plan to manage your MS, it's also a good idea to come up with a household management plan that outlines duties and responsibilities and clarifies how you're going to look at them from now on.

A good way to start is by learning how to simplify tasks. Reorganize your home so that you feel a certain ease in living. Come up with a chart that organizes chores and requires everyone to share the workload. Take a look at your budget and see if you can afford to get some help cleaning bathrooms or mowing the lawn. Prioritizing tasks can help you figure out where you need to direct your time and energy.

One of the most important tasks in keeping it together is prioritizing time with your family members. Many people with MS have reported difficulty in keeping perspective; MS can easily take over a family, so you'll want to establish quality time with your loved ones in an MS-free zone. Even if some of the activities you once enjoyed are off limits, the quality of your time together doesn't have to change. If hiking or skiing are no longer possible, a beautiful ride in the country can be a nice way to enjoy nature. You want to balance the needs of everyone in the family while leaving a little room for the realities of MS to coincide. Mom or Dad can read a good book in the ski lodge and have lunch ready for everyone at noon rather than having the whole family give up skiing. There is no shortage of ideas to help you adapt—it just takes creativity and flexibility on everyone's part.

Alert

Parents must also be careful to nurture their own relationship. Setting aside time to spend alone together is crucial. The connection between two parents is fundamental to the rest of the family, so you'll want to schedule quality time with your spouse, such as a weekly movie or dinner night. Dressing up and leaving the last load of laundry behind can go a long way in helping you remember that you're a couple.

Parenting with MS

Studies show that kids who have a parent with MS tend to adapt and do well in life, so if you have concerns about what sort of effect MS is going to have in the life of your children, you can breathe a bit easier knowing that. In fact, kids who deal with health issues in their family tend to be more compassionate and sensitive toward others.

Being a parent with MS has extra challenges, whether it's learning how to more effectively manage your time, restructuring family activities, or answering difficult questions—inevitably you'll deal with some tough issues. But families that tackle difficult times grow closer to one another and tend to learn very quickly what's most important in life.

Explaining Your Symptoms

Children don't have a hard time understanding visible symptoms such as weakness or difficulty walking, but the invisible ones may be harder to explain. If you decide to skip out on a family outing because of fatigue, for example, it may be difficult for your child to understand the reason behind it because it's something he can't see. To prevent misinterpretation of your actions, it's important to educate your kids about the reality of MS early on. You don't want a temporary lack of involvement to send the wrong message.

Essential

Being creative in your parenting approach is essential. Instead of heading to the movies when you're tired, you can cuddle on the couch and read a story together. Find some great shopping sites online and take a shopping spree with your daughter. The key to good parenting is to stay active and involved in your child's life and find unique opportunities to spend time together.

Redefining Parenthood

So many of the roles we play as parents are culturally determined: Dad plays ball in the yard; Mom does the school shopping and folds the clothes. Showing your love through physical endeavors is something you may not have given any thought to. Sometimes having MS causes people to redefine their roles as parents and what it means to be a parent, especially when there are activities they can no longer participate in. One father explained how he reinvented the game of football with his sons: When his symptoms progressed and made mobility difficult, he was the quarterback on the field and remained stationary, tossing the ball to his sons. He found a creative way to enjoy the things they used to do—with some modification. Not being able to perform some of the physical activities with their children can also lead people with MS to harbor feelings of isolation and sadness, so it's important to get the toolbox out and find other ways to enjoy your time together. Find a used tandem bike or buy a motorized scooter to enjoy evening walks with your family. The point is to adapt by being creative.

Finding Help

Even in the best of situations, parenting can be difficult. Don't be afraid to seek out the help of support groups, mental health professionals, or family members.

If you're having problems with fatigue, call on a family member or friend to take your son to the ball game. Families that have a strong support network tend to manage better, so rally the troops when you need help. You might find that your friends and family are happy to find a way they can be there for you.

Alert

> Children spend an average of 900 hours a year in school, but spend more than 1,500 hours a year watching television, according to the A.C. Nielsen Co. The average child will spend more than thirty hours per week parked in front of a TV. While the "electronic babysitter" can be helpful on days when you're extra tired, have some other tricks up your sleeve that will encourage your kids to be more creative with their time.

It's Not All about MS

It's tempting to blame everything that happens on MS, but keep in mind that teenagers are ornery, young children can be difficult, and all families cope with their share of hard times. You might want to check on your family members' emotional health from time to time and not automatically assume that any unusual behavior or problems that arise are caused by having MS. Kids go through all kinds of hardships with friends, school, and self-esteem on their way through life. Some parents with MS feel badly that their children have to cope with an illness in the home, but remember: Good parenting is imperative for all children, and good old-fashioned discipline and teaching responsibility are important. There are some great parenting books on the market; a good family therapist can help you deal with parenting issues as well.

Family Trips

Traveling with the family has never been easy, but now's the time to find ways to simplify! You don't have to give up your yearly treks to the campground or Disney World if you initiate some good planning strategies. In fact, any cherished family routines should be encouraged when possible. Making new memories is an important part of family life. Make sure you talk to your neurologist before making plans; she may have some good advice or concerns to share with you, too.

Essential

If you're looking for tips when traveling with young kids, check out *The Rough Guide to Travel with Babies & Young Children*. The book includes a variety of tips, including coping with road trips and plane travel, health concerns, entertaining kids on the road, and cultural issues. You'll find some great ways to save energy—and your sanity.

Travel Tips

Before you head off to Yosemite, there are a few things you'll need to think about, such as what to do with your MS medications and how you can make traveling a bit easier for yourself. Here are a few good tips to consider:

- Traveling with disease-modifying therapy medication can be tricky these days, so be sure to plan ahead. A doctor's note explaining that you have MS is useful in certain situations, especially getting through security with needles in your carry-on luggage. Keep your meds in their original containers. Bring enough medication along to last you an extra week in case your stay is extended. Bring along the original prescription label and a photo ID that matches the name on the prescription.
- Pack all of your medications in a carry-on bag. If any of your medications need to be refrigerated, ice packs in an insulated lunch pouch do a good job.
- Your neurologist may give you a prescription for steroids in case you have an exacerbation while traveling. This is a good thing to consider requesting before you leave.
- Use a travel agent to ensure safe travel. If mobility is an issue, a good travel agent can help you arrange for accessible flights and hotels. You don't want to leave anything to chance. There are travel agents that specialize in travel for folks with disabilities, too.
- Flying is fraught with its own discomforts: cancelled planes, long delays, and layovers. Be realistic when booking your flight. Two layovers can make for a long day. Request an aisle seat so you can stand up and stretch or use the bathroom when you need to.
- If you're headed somewhere new, research your destination. Know the average temperature for the time of year in which you're traveling. Some countries have laws pertaining to disability, but many do not. It's important to know what to expect. Make sure your hotel has air conditioning if you're headed somewhere warm.

- Plan your activities carefully. Don't put yourself in a situation that you can't get out of, such as sitting in a boat under a blazing sun for eight hours. Bring along a commercial cooling vest, wear light-colored clothing, and try to plan your trip during the coolest season of the year, if possible.
- Use your time wisely. It's important to schedule rest breaks during the day to conserve your energy. Have a "Top Five" list of the things you'd most like to do on vacation so you're not tempted to plan too many activities.

Families that live with MS sometimes have more than their share of issues to contend with, but education, support, and planning can ease a lot of your concerns. Kids are known to be resilient, but careful attention to their emotional health is a good way to assess their well-being and keep the family on track. Creative parenting is your greatest resource; it's one way to overcome some of the limitations some folks contend with and provides you with the opportunity to find new ways to do old things.

CHAPTER 17

MS and Real Life

SINCE MS IS often diagnosed right in the middle of the prime career and family-building years, the questions you have are important ones: Should I stay on this career path? Should I get married? Can I plan a family? While many couples can and do have families after a diagnosis of MS, it's important to ask the right questions and get a handle on the issues, both big and small, surrounding childbirth, family life, and the tasks of daily living.

Pregnancy: Your Questions and Concerns

Your ability to get pregnant does not seem to be affected by MS, so that's the good news. Women with MS conceive at the same rate as other women who do not have MS. Additionally, research has shown that pregnancy and childbirth don't have any long-term negative effects on most women with MS. It's uncommon for expectant mothers to experience a worsening of symptoms while they're pregnant. In fact, for many women with MS, pregnancy seems to offer some protection from exacerbations. Here are some other things to keep in mind:

- Labor for a woman with MS is usually handled in the same way as it is for other women. In general, moms with MS deliver their babies like everyone else.
- Expectant women with MS are more susceptible to other health problems, such as fatigue, urinary tract infections, and constipation. An obstetrician may suggest certain precautions, such as using a stool softener to counter constipation, having regular urine cultures to detect possible infections, or changing MS medications.
- Research shows no elevated risk of exacerbations caused by breastfeeding. Certain medications may be off limits, and some mothers may be too tired to breastfeed. It's a personal choice that you should explore with your MS specialist.
- The risk that your baby will someday develop MS is about 1 to 5 percent. Although MS is not a directly inherited disorder, genetic factors are thought to increase the risk of developing MS in some individuals.
- Women with MS can have healthy, full-term babies. Research shows that there is no increased risk for miscarriages.

People are often surprised to find that pregnancy is a viable option for women with MS and that there appear to be few—if any—physical implications beyond an increased risk of relapse following childbirth. The challenge comes from thinking things through—putting the what-ifs into play and problem-solving potential issues such as disease progression or physical limitation.

Essential

Since you can't be sure how you'll be feeling two or three years down the road, it's often difficult to think ahead, so a good rule of thumb is to imagine what you'd do in certain situations, such as losing or leaving a job or having problems with mobility or fatigue. Problem solving before problems arise is a good stress-management strategy.

The Planning Process

Deciding to start a family is a big decision for any couple, but for those living with MS, there are a number of considerations to take into account. Practical issues such as financial security and employment come into play, as well as long-term considerations such as how many children you'd like to have and how MS may affect your parenting ability. While the statistics are in your favor, it's important to be cognizant that you may be the exception and have a relapse following pregnancy. The truth is, in order to make a well-informed decision you have to hope for the best and plan for the worst. You have to troubleshoot any potential problems and figure out now how you'd handle them.

 Alert

> In the postpartum stage, research indicates that exacerbations increase in nearly 30 percent of cases, so your chances of having a relapse after giving birth are somewhat greater. You're most at risk in the first three to six months after you've given birth. Further, women who are experiencing active MS before their pregnancy may be more at risk for having a relapse following pregnancy.

There are a few things that need serious consideration before starting a family:

- **Your financial status.** Diapers and nursery school are only the tip of the iceberg. Financial security also includes college planning, health and life insurance, and job security. Before deciding to start a family, you should take a good look at your finances and troubleshoot any potential problems, such as a partner who might decide to leave the work force early or the possibility that you'll change careers. A financial planner can help you get your financial house in order.

- **Timing.** The disease-modifying therapies are not approved for use during pregnancy or breastfeeding, so you'll have to stop the medication two to three months before you become pregnant. If you decide to breastfeed, you won't be able to resume the DMTs until you're through nursing your baby.
- **The numbers.** You may have once imagined that you'd have a house full of kids, but it's time to reconsider the number. Five children will be five times the demand on your time and energy and you don't want to spread yourself too thinly.
- **Support.** Take a good look at your support network and see if that helps you in the decision-making process. People who have oodles of relatives on hand may feel more secure knowing they have people they can depend on if things get tough. If you think you could use a bit more support, be proactive in developing a network. Parenting groups give you opportunities to meet other parents. Neighbors and friends are a good source of support, too. You may want to look into hiring some help as well, such as a babysitter who can give you a few hours' break on a Saturday afternoon.

Alert

If you were recently diagnosed, your doctor may want you to consider postponing pregnancy for a year or two until you've gotten a handle on things and you've given your DMT a chance to kick in. Your MS specialist will have valuable insight, so make an appointment to talk to him during the baby-planning process. The timing of having a family is a deeply personal issue, but one you need to carefully explore.

The First Year

The first year of a baby's life is exhausting for parents and you'll be hard pressed to find anyone to tell you any differently! Good planning and realistic expectations can help you over the humps, though.

Researchers aren't exactly sure why women are at increased risk of experiencing a relapse after giving birth, but they theorize it may have something to do with postpartum hormonal fluctuations. When you add in a lack of sleep and a whole host of new tasks and chores, it's easy to see how new parents can feel drained.

Be sure to call in the troops after you've given birth. Having a family member to support you those first few weeks is invaluable, especially if it's someone who has experience with newborns. Being able to take a hot shower or a short nap is not only wonderful, but important to your health and well-being.

Have your friends or neighbors pledge their support before the baby is born. In other words, schedule rest and relaxation for yourself before you need it. Beyond your support network, you may want to limit guests for the first few weeks to give yourself a chance to recuperate.

If you're planning on going back to work, take as much maternity leave as possible. Remember, you'll be doing double duty when you leave your job each day to juggle the responsibility of home and children. You'll want to use your break from work as a time to connect with your child, but also to establish a good health regimen. Your goal will also be to regain your strength.

Enlist the support of your spouse or someone else you trust to help you with daily tasks, including nighttime feedings. If you're breastfeeding, learning to use a breast pump will add some flexibility to your schedule.

Good planning and strategizing will go a long way in helping you to manage the challenges of starting a family.

MS and Relationships

You've just met someone you're interested in and when you're deciding how long to wait until you call her again (not more than one day!), you also wonder how—and if—to broach the subject of MS. Do you get it over with right away or wait until it's absolutely necessary? There's no right or wrong answer here, but there are certain factors you may want to consider when thinking it through.

It's All about Self-Esteem

You've heard it before, but it's true that MS is only part of who you are. There's a whole lot more to you than your diagnosis; your memories, skills, hobbies, interests, and feelings are also part of who you are. You'll want to make it your goal to be comfortable with yourself, to believe wholeheartedly in your value as a human being and potential partner to someone you love. This can take some time. Learning to live with MS is a process of self-discovery. Sometimes you have to test your mettle, assess your strengths and weaknesses, and go the course for a while until you come to a place of acceptance. There may not be a magical day when you wake up and feel perfectly comfortable in your own shoes; it's more a process than it is a moment. But you'll know when you're there. You'll feel pride in your ability to overcome obstacles; you'll see MS as one piece of the puzzle that makes up your complexity rather than a hurdle you're constantly trying to jump over.

Essential

Pay close attention to your self-esteem and make sure you take care of all of you. Work at your career and your hobbies. Cultivate the special parts of you that make you unique. When you feel comfortable and at peace with yourself, you will inevitably reflect that to others.

In his book, *Healing the Shame That Binds You*, John Bradshaw says: "Total self-love and acceptance is the only foundation for happiness and the love of others. Without total self-love and acceptance, we are doomed to the enervating task of creating false selves."

Self-acceptance means loving yourself as you are, including all of your thoughts, feelings, and actions. It also means showing yourself some compassion. Experts say most people are kinder to others than they are to themselves, so pay attention to your own internal dialogue. Are you kind and patient with yourself or is your inner dialogue critical and overbearing? It's important to turn the negative thoughts about yourself into positive ones. If you want to change your life, change your thinking.

You are solely responsible for your own happiness. Knowing this, you can start to pay attention to your needs and desires and make sure you are doing all you can to nurture your happiness quotient. Self-assessment is important here; you'll have to know what makes you happy first and then find ways to include those things in your life. Since MS may sometimes limit your choices, find alternate ways to do the things you love.

Take Care of Yourself

As children, many people are taught that the purpose of life is to take care of others. They learned to "behave" and to be "selfless." Consequently, there are people who have no idea how to nurture and care for themselves. Give yourself permission to be your own best friend. Take good care of your emotional and physical health.

So, what does self-esteem have to do with dating and MS? While most everyone feels unhappy with themselves from time to time, people with MS and other chronic illnesses are prone to feelings of low self-worth and a lack of self-confidence. Believing that their body has somehow failed them, not feeling as if they've adequately reached their goals in life, dealing with financial difficulties and intermittent symptoms—these are some of the issues people with MS may face that take a toll on their emotional health.

When it comes to dating and relationships, feeling good about who you are is one of the most important aspects of attracting and sustaining a healthy relationship. You want to cultivate a strong sense of individual worth that does not rely on others for its nourishment. High self-esteem is not only important to your well-being, it is also attractive to others.

Keep in mind that low self-esteem can also signal depression, so it's important to get help if you're feeling low for more than a week or two.

Sharing Your Diagnosis

Figuring out the right time to tell your family, friends, employer, or date about your MS is a little tricky. You're trying to balance your right to privacy with your need to be honest and forthright. A good rule of thumb is this: When you believe the other person has a need to know, and you feel comfortable doing so, then go ahead and explain your situation. While that may seem straightforward, things can get a little murky. For example, one woman with MS never felt comfortable sharing the fact that she had MS with a man she'd grown close to, and in the end, it cost her the relationship. Mind you, he didn't leave because she had MS; she eventually stopped calling him back because she felt uncomfortable hiding it for so long. And here's where self-esteem plays a big role: you have to be comfortable with who you are in order to share yourself with someone else. Learn to trust your instincts and not your fears when it comes to disclosure while dating.

Alert

It isn't necessary to divulge your MS on a first date. First dates are for getting to know someone else, and deciding if you are interested in getting closer to that person. If you don't have a second date, nothing has been lost by not sharing your diagnosis.

It's when you start spending real time with someone else that you may feel obligated to be more up front. You don't want to be accused of being deceitful, although in reality you are attempting to protect yourself by letting that person get to know you before you share something that may change his mind about having a relationship with you. There's a balance you must strike between putting your best foot forward and divulging the intimate details of your life. Waiting too long can also cost you more: if the person decides against going further in the relationship, you may already be emotionally invested and have a lot more to lose. You may also find that you favor the speedier route: tell the other person as soon as possible (maybe even the first date). Better to know his reaction right away before investing anything into the relationship.

Only you can decide what feels comfortable, but a little planning can go a long way. Be ready to answer some questions about what MS is and how it affects you. And since MS is commonly misunderstood, be ready to debunk some myths—most commonly the myth that MS always leads to physical limitation or disability. Talking openly and honestly can help put the other person at ease. In the end, it's up to him to decide whether he chooses to continue the relationship. If things don't go the way you had hoped, try not to invest too much of yourself in the outcome. Know that you can and will survive rejection and that risk, after all, is part of the dating game for all singles.

Try to keep in mind that people with MS do date, marry, and have families all the time. You may find that certain people are more open to the idea of dating someone with MS than others, and so it becomes a matter of finding the right person, someone who understands you and sees you for who you are.

MS and the Holidays

There's nothing like the winter holidays to bring out the fanatics in all of us, whether you've always made thirty dozen cookies, had the biggest holiday party on the block, or vowed to shop until you drop. Even the heartiest among us have their limits—and setting limits is a good way to maneuver through the holiday crunch when stress is at a maximum and energy is scarce.

Living with MS, as you've learned, requires balance, and the holidays can really put your simplification skills to the test. It's good to develop strategies that will allow you to manage the season with a sense of ease and grace.

Make Lists

Checklists are a good way to prioritize your tasks; in fact, they're a great way to get rid of tasks. When you make your lists, go through them again and decide what you can cut out this year. Do you really need to adhere to every single tradition? Can you just buy eggnog this year instead of making it from scratch? Can you pick names with your siblings instead of shopping for everyone? What can you leave off your list that will make life easier?

Delegate Tasks

When you hear "But, Mom, we've always made cookies from scratch," you might want to see how important that tradition is to the rest of the family by handing them the flour. Because you've decided you can't do it all, it's time to get everyone else in the corner with the scotch tape and scissors. Learning to delegate is a skill used by CEOs and mothers worldwide.

Revamp Your Expectations

Christmas brings out perfectionists like nothing else. People often have a picture in their minds about what their celebrations should be like, often cultivated from childhood memories. Learning to rethink your celebrations is a good idea. Instead of imagining the holidays as a time of busy, chaotic festivity, perhaps it might serve you to see it as a time of solitude and reflection, where you cuddle up with your kids with a cup of cocoa and watch Christmas movies, or you spend time helping those who are less fortunate. Not everyone dashes through the holidays at lightning speed; some prefer to see it as a time to relax and enjoy special time with their family.

Try Some Time Savers

Figure out ways to cut corners rather than doing things the way you've always done them. Here are some tips:

- Shop online. Reputable stores and online sites are careful to protect your security, so you can shop online without concern. There's something great about clicking a mouse on a desired gift and having it show up at your door a few days later—wrapped.

- Send e-mails instead of holiday cards. There are some great websites that allow you to add pictures and your own sentiments to electronic cards. Try *www.smilebox.com.*
- Have a cookie exchange party where everyone goes home with a selection of treats that others have baked and contributed.
- Have your favorite restaurant make your side dishes, your local grocery store cook your turkey, or the bakery make your pies. This might sting a little at first, but you might find it takes a lot of the stress out of the big holiday dinner or other gatherings.
- Have everyone contribute a dish for holiday dinners or parties.
- Gift certificates make great gifts, especially if you know which stores your recipients enjoy.
- Take the word "should" out of Christmas and do only what you enjoy or feel capable of doing.

Keep in mind that the stress of the holidays may cause some people to neglect their usual self-care routine—something you want to avoid. Pare down your obligations if you find yourself falling into that trap.

Flu Shots and Other Vaccinations

Cases of influenza are common during the winter months, and the flu vaccine has gone a long way in relieving the discomfort for millions of yearly sufferers. Although there used to be some confusion about whether or not people with MS should get a shot each year, recent studies indicate that flu shots are safe and, generally, are reasonable for people with RRMS. Here's what you need to know:

A 1997 study looked for possible links between the influenza vaccination and MS relapses and found that people with RRMS who were injected with the vaccine did not have more relapses than those who were injected with a placebo. On the other hand, studies indicate that the flu may provoke an MS attack. In summary, the flu vaccination does not appear to cause attacks, but the flu itself may cause attacks. Experts still advise you to discuss the issue with your doctor before deciding whether or not to get the vaccine.

Who Should Not Get the Shot?

Anyone with an active or unstable neurological condition, including people with MS who are having a relapse, should avoid the influenza vaccine or postpone it until four to six weeks after the onset of relapse. Also, flu vaccination should probably be avoided by people with MS who have a history of attacks that appear to have been provoked by the flu vaccine. There are other situations in which people are advised not to get the shot:

- Infants under the age of six months
- Anyone who is allergic to or has had an anaphylactic hypersensitivity to eggs or egg products
- Anyone who has had an allergic or anaphylactic reaction to a previous flu vaccination
- Anyone who is actively unwell at the time of the vaccination (high fever and chills); they should postpone receiving the flu vaccine until symptoms have become better

In a nutshell, researchers say that flu shots are safe for folks with RRMS and can prevent infections that can trigger or worsen MS symptoms. In the past, some patients and their doctors worried that the vaccine could cause a relapse by triggering an immune response, but experts say that's unlikely. Patients with other forms of the disease or with high disease activity should talk to their doctor about whether to vaccinate.

Other Vaccinations

Based on current evidence, it appears that hepatitis B, tetanus, measles, and rubella (German measles) vaccinations are safe for people with MS and are not associated with an increased risk for the development of MS or optic neuritis. The hepatitis B vaccine in particular was in question as to whether or not it caused or worsened MS as well as other neurological conditions, but studies found no links between the two. A 2001 panel studying the issue recommended that people with MS have access to life- saving vaccines and that they use the Center for Disease Control guidelines (*www.cdc.gov*) for information on vaccines. Other recommendations include:

- People who have received immune globulin preparation in the past three months should not receive live attenuated virus vaccines, such as varicella or MMR (measles, mumps, and rubella).
- People on therapies that suppress the immune system (immunosuppressants), such as mitoxantrone, natalizumab (tysabri) azathioprine, methotrexate, cyclophosphamide and/or chronic corticosteroid therapy should not receive live attenuated vaccines. A person with a suppressed immune system would be at greater risk for developing the disease.

Live attenuated vaccines contain viruses that have been altered so they can't cause disease. Viruses are weakened by growing them in such a way that their disease-causing ability is decreased.

Beat the Heat

Somewhere between 60 and 80 percent of people with MS have intolerance to heat, where a rise in internal or external temperature can temporarily increase symptoms. A hot and humid environment, a fever during illness, exercising, sunbathing—even hot showers and baths—can cause your symptoms to flare.

These temporary changes result from an increase in your core body temperature. Even as little as to one-quarter to one-half degree in temperature rise can cause you problems. A buildup of heat slows down nerve transmission, causing symptoms to worsen.

While this certainly doesn't bode well for your summer plans, the good news is that these symptoms are "phantom" symptoms and are not typically causing any type of permanent tissue damage. The symptoms decrease once the source of heat is removed.

So, what are the symptoms of heat intolerance? It shouldn't be hard to identify, but here are a few of the typical symptoms you may experience:

- Fatigue may increase as well as tremors and cognitive difficulties.
- Some people notice that their vision becomes blurred when they get overheated; this is known as Uhthoff's phenomenon.
- Other chronic symptoms—those that are familiar to you on a day-to-day basis—may also increase in the heat.
- Some people report swelling of the legs or feet.

Tips on Cooling Down

You don't have to stop doing the things you enjoy but you may have to change the way you do certain things. For example, taking a shower rather than a bath and decreasing the temperature might help. Everyone has his own set point for heat intolerance, so you might have to experiment to see what works for you.

- Drink plenty of fluids. Water or diluted fruit juices are best.
- When going outdoors consider taking frozen items, such as frozen lollipops or ice cubes.

- Try to stay indoors in an air conditioned environment on really hot and humid days.
- Decrease your core body temperature before engaging in an activity by taking a cool shower. This also helps some people with fatigue.
- Invest in equipment that helps you manage the heat, such as cooling vests, mister fans, and cooling gel wristbands.
- Eat cool foods. Salads, sandwiches, fruit, cold soups, raw veggies—these are all good cooling foods.
- Take a swim. Pools with water temperature under 85°F are ideal for exercising or just cooling down.
- Get "the tag." You might want to apply for a disabled parking placard even if you are able to walk. Walking through a parking lot on the hottest day of the year may convince you that this is a worthwhile venture.
- Window tinting may be expensive, but it can pay for itself in a few years by lowering your air conditioning bills. Window tinting is not just for cars anymore!

There are numerous ways to keep cool in hot weather, so be sure to get creative when rethinking outdoor activities. You don't want to stop doing those activities that bring you fulfillment.

Fact

The Multiple Sclerosis Association of America (MSAA) has a Cooling Equipment Distribution Program to get cooling products to people with MS that need them but cannot afford them. They have a variety of cooling products, such as bandanas, vests, collars—even cooling suits. For more information, visit *www.msassociation.org/programs/cooling* or call 1-800-532-7667.

In fact, real life with MS is about solutions—finding creative ways to get around the hurdles that MS presents to you, whether it's starting a family, traveling to Europe, or hiking in the summer months. It's also about letting go of those things that no longer serve you, and accepting those that will make your life easier, whether it's letting someone else prepare the turkey this year or simply learning to accept help from others. The truth is that managing MS requires you to be in the driver's seat and firmly in control. The quality of your life depends on it.

CHAPTER 18

The Future with MS

THERE IS GOOD reason to be hopeful about the future of multiple sclerosis treatment. Research is accelerating, new treatments are being studied, and the mysteries surrounding the disease are being steadily unveiled. The NMSS is currently spending $440 million annually on more than 400 MS investigations, and MS is being studied on a wide array of fronts. According to the NMSS, there are more potential therapies in the pipeline for MS than ever before.

Oral Therapies

Oral therapies that can one day replace injectable therapies are eagerly anticipated by people with MS who would like to avoid the discomfort of needles and injection-site reactions. Experts anticipate that oral therapies will greatly increase the number of people who get on the DMTs early and stay on their chosen therapies. Here are a few oral therapies that look promising:

- Oral laquinimod (Teva Pharmaceuticals) is an immunomodulating drug being studied for those with relapsing-remitting MS. It is administered once daily.

- Fingolimod (also known as FTY720) (Novartis Pharmaceuticals) is an oral drug that binds to a docking site on immune cells, preventing them from leaving the lymph nodes and thereby preventing them from attacking the brain and spinal cord. It is under study in about 2,000 people with RRMS in Europe and North America. It is administered once daily.
- Mylinax (oral cladribine) (EMD, Serono and IVAX) is a daily, orally administered disease-modifying treatment for RRMS. Mylinax interferes with the activity and the proliferation of certain white blood cells, particularly lymphocytes, which are involved in the pathological process of MS.
- Teriflunomide (Sanofi-Aventis) is a daily, orally administered disease-modifying treatment for RRMS and SPMS. It is thought to prevent damage of the nervous system by T cells, one form of immune cells.
- BG-12 (oral fumarate) (Biogen Idec) is an oral fumarate for RRMS. It regulates the immune system and may also protect cells from injury.

Researchers agree that an effective oral treatment would be a significant breakthrough in the management of MS. The therapies will be taken in an oral form, eliminating the need for injection training and creating ease in administering the drug. Some of these drugs are currently in Phase III trials (the last trial phase before applying for FDA approval), which generally last two to three years.

Fact

Since women seem to have added protection against relapse during pregnancy, research is focusing on estriol, a female sex hormone, which is believed to suppress the immune system in women with MS during pregnancy. Current research is teaming a pill form of estriol with Copaxone (Teva Pharmaceuticals).

Therapies for Progressive MS

Research is targeting drugs for the progressive forms of MS, for which there are very few treatments at the moment. There are several treatments for PPMS and SPMS in the pipeline:

- MBP8298 (BioMS Medical Corp.) is currently being studied for progressive forms of MS. It is a synthetic fragment of a protein found in myelin.
- Cytoxan (cyclophosphamide), an immunosuppressive drug usually used to treat cancer, is currently being studied for its effectiveness in treating SPMS.
- Lamictal (lamotrigine) (Glaxo-SmithKline) is an oral drug currently used to prevent seizures in people with epilepsy. It is currently being studied for SPMS.

Although the tide is turning, historically the emphasis of research has been placed on relapsing-remitting MS because the greatest percentages of people are diagnosed with this form, and because it is easier to measure and observe changes in RRMS. Also, the inflammation found in RRMS provides a specific target for treatment.

Primary progressive patients appear to have less or a different type of inflammation, and so far, inflammation has been easier to treat. All six of the FDA-approved disease-modifying therapies target inflammation caused by the immune system's attack on the CNS. They are most effective for individuals with RRMS, with limited effectiveness for some individuals with SPMS. Drugs that target inflammation do not seem to have much effect on those with non-relapsing forms of MS.

Research, however, is accelerating, and people with progressive forms of MS have reason to look ahead and be optimistic.

The Future of Symptom Relief

Until a cure is found, much of the focus in treating MS will be on managing and improving symptoms. Here are a few of the treatments on the horizon for MS symptoms:

- **Fatigue.** Researchers have found that people with MS who take four regular aspirin tablets per day reduced fatigue compared to those who took the placebo. Further study is under way. People interested in this approach should discuss this with their physician, since long-term use of high-dose aspirin may cause side effects.
- **Pain.** Sativex (GW Pharmaceuticals), a drug derived from the cannabis plant, is being studied for effectiveness in relieving pain and other MS-related symptoms. It is administered as a spray directly into the mouth and is approved for use in Canada.
- **Spasticity.** Studies are under way to test the effectiveness and safety of Sativex and other marijuana-related therapies as a way to relieve spasticity in MS.
- **Mobility.** Researchers are looking at a new rehabilitative technique called *locomotor training*, which is an activity- based therapy that attempts to retrain the brain to remember the pattern of walking. In MS, an individual is assisted by a robotic device that moves the legs.
- **Bladder function.** Scientists have developed a "bladder pacemaker" that has helped people with urinary incontinence in preliminary trials. The pacemaker, is surgically implanted, and controlled by a hand-held unit that allows the patient to electrically stimulate the nerves that control bladder function.

Researchers are also trying to identify subtypes of MS based on MRI findings, specific proteins in the blood or spinal fluid, and specific genes. It is hoped that these subtypes may respond particularly well to specific kinds of therapies. This type of work may lead to MS treatment that is "tailored" to the individual in the future.

Stem Cell Research

Recent studies have shown that adult brain cells can repair the damage caused by immune cells in the central nervous system. Here's how it works: Stem cells found in an adult brain have the remarkable ability to turn into many different kinds of cells, and when these stem cells are injected into mice with an MS-like disease, the cells travel to the damaged nerves and repair them. Even though testing has only been conducted on mice, it's an exciting breakthrough. Here's what they've found so far:

- The brain stem cells zero in on damaged nerves.
- They replace nerve cells killed by disease.
- They help rebuild the myelin coating on the outside of nerve fibers.
- The mice in the study improved from the disease.

Keep in mind that the treatment doesn't halt the immune system attack that characterizes MS, and, for now, research is focusing on stem cells as a possible approach for repair or replacement.

Blood Test to Diagnose MS

Scientists believe that it may be possible one day to use a simple blood test to diagnose MS. People with relapsing-remitting MS may have a distinct pattern of proteins in their blood that may be detectable with a simple test. A quick diagnosis would enable people with MS to begin receiving support and treatment early on, thus alleviating the stress that often comes with the diagnostic process.

Statins and MS Research

The use of statins to treat MS has been generating some excitement. Statins, such as the drug Lipitor, are usually used to lower cholesterol. Researchers have discovered that they may also be effective in treating autoimmune illnesses. Statins appear to lower the number of new lesions in the brain from MS by decreasing inflammation. Research shows that patients taking statins with their standard drug regimen develop less nerve cell damage over time than those patients on standard therapy alone. Researchers predict that statins may be used to enhance current treatments for MS and may offer a means of preventing progression of the disease as they reduce the inflammation that causes nerve cell damage. Although research so far is encouraging, further work is needed in this area to determine whether statins are actually safe and effective in MS.

Genetic Research

Genetic research into the causes of MS uses cutting-edge technology and allows researchers to identify the genes that cause or predispose a person to the disease. It will also help science to target new treatment strategies and perhaps isolate the cause.

Three recent large-scale genetic studies uncovered new genetic variations connected with MS, specifically the interleukin-7 receptor alpha, which may lead to impaired immune responses. These findings have led researchers to study the drug daclizumab, also known by the trade name Zenapax, a drug used to prevent kidney transplant rejection. A clinical trial of patients with multiple sclerosis who did not respond to interferon alone found that adding the human antibody daclizumab improved patient outcome.

Essential

Experimental allergic encephalomyelitis (EAE) is an animal model of MS, usually studied in mice. It is brought on by artificially triggering the immune system to attack myelin. EAE is not exactly the same as MS, but studies of the various forms of EAE are thought to provide some insight into the nature of MS and potential treatments.

Remyelination

There is a great deal of interest in pursuing treatments that will reverse the MS-induced damage to myelin and oligodendrocytes, the cells that make and maintain myelin in the central nervous system. Research has found that oligodendrocytes may proliferate and form new myelin after an attack. Studies of animal models indicate that some types of antibodies may accelerate remyelination.

Cytokines

Research has allowed science to study the inner workings of the immune system and the functioning of cytokines, which are proteins produced by T cells and other immune cells. Scientists hope to discover how they can block harmful cytokines and increase the production of protective cytokines in MS. Two drugs are currently being studied to this end: rolipram has been shown to reduce levels of several destructive cytokines in animal models of MS, and interleukin-4 (IL-4) may be able to influence developing T cells to become protective rather than harmful.

Question

Have scientists created an MS vaccine?
Early results from several studies looked promising, but it appears investigators have a long way to go before their hopes for an MS vaccine can come to fruition. One form of vaccination treatment involves extracting cells from each patient, purifying them and growing them in a culture before inactivating and chemically altering them.

Participating in a Clinical Trial

Clinical trials test potential treatments in human volunteers to see if they should be used in the general population. They're an important part of product discovery and development and are required by the

FDA before a new product can be brought to the market. The federal government has established strict regulations and guidelines for clinical research to protect participants from unreasonable risks. Although efforts are made to control risks, they can't be completely eliminated, so it's important to get a handle on the process and the risks that may be involved. Before deciding whether or not to participate in a clinical trial, it's useful to understand the process that a potential new drug or therapy undergoes before it is approved and marketed.

Only 1 in every 5,000 compounds survives the process of FDA approval in the United States, while the cost of developing a drug averages $897 million in a ten- to fifteen-year period. Clearly, all new therapies must weave their way through a stringent process before they are brought to market. Here's a brief outline of the process:

1. **Preclinical trials.** In this phase, potential therapies are tested in the laboratory and on animals to determine toxicity and side effects. After each stage, the sponsor of the new therapy meets with the FDA to determine their next steps and establish the parameters for future trials.

2. **Clinical evaluation.** In this phase, the sponsoring company approaches the FDA with the results from the preclinical studies and files an Investigational New Drug application. They also submit a proposal to study the dosage and safety in humans.

3. **Phase I—Safety.** Dosing for future trials and safety is assessed. In Phase I treatment trials, a small number of volunteer patients (usually between fifteen and thirty) are given the experimental treatment in gradually larger doses to test for any side effects or complications. The researchers conducting the trial will also try to determine what a safe dose would be and how it should be given.

4. **Phase II—Safety and Efficacy.** In this phase, studies are conducted to test for therapeutic effect as well as safety. The studies are usually larger at this point, with 40 to 300 participants. Several studies may be carried out in this

phase so that the therapy can be studied in a variety of patient populations.

5. **Phase III—Controlled Safety and Efficacy.** In this phase, larger patient populations are used to confirm the beneficial effect from Phase II trials and to continue to monitor side effects. These trials can involve hundreds to thousands of people. The product is also compared to other treatment options or used in combination with other treatment approaches.

6. **Regulatory filing.** In this stage, the company submits an application for marketing approval, along with all the data collected in the trials. The FDA has at least six months to review a "priority" application (drugs for a life-threatening need) and ten months for a standard application. Final approval can take up to two years.

7. **Phase IV—FDA Approval and Post-Approval Monitoring.** Doctors can now prescribe the new drug, although the sponsoring company must continue to monitor any adverse side effects and report them to the FDA.

8. **Manufacturing.** The FDA regulates the manufacturing of drugs by, in some cases, testing several lots of drugs prior to marketing as well as inspecting manufacturing facilities and requiring companies to keep manufacturing records.

Which treatment each participant receives in these studies is determined by a process called *randomization*, where the treatments are randomly selected by a computer.

Essential

Phase II and III of a clinical trial often involve a control group, where one group is given the test drug and another is given a standardized treatment or a placebo, depending on the study. The control group provides the basis of comparison for the new treatment.

Studies are often blind studies or double-blind studies. A double-blind study is one in which neither the researcher nor the participants know who is receiving the experimental treatment and who is receiving the standard treatment or placebo. Blinding is done to ensure that neither the participant nor the researchers' expectations can influence the results.

Who Can Participate?

Each clinical trial has a set of inclusion and exclusion rules. These rules are designed to safely test the effectiveness of a treatment and to ensure the safety of the participants. In a trial for MS, for example, inclusion might be limited to people with a certain form of the disease, such as relapsing-remitting. A clinical trial may exclude people with certain medical conditions or those taking specific medications.

Certain tests and procedures are carried out on participants before the trial begins. These tests determine eligibility and establish the overall health of the patient and can include blood tests or neurological examinations, for example. Tests are also used to measure the effect of the treatment. These tests are often given before, during, and after the treatment to determine if the treatment improves the condition being studied compared to the control group. Clinical trials often require more tests and visits to doctors than would be required with standard treatment. For example, participants may be required to have regular MRIs, neurological exams, or blood tests.

All trials must follow a protocol, which is a set of rules on which the study is based. The protocol describes who is eligible to participate, the length of the study, details of the schedule and procedures, and any medications that will be involved, including the dosage prescribed.

The term *informed consent* refers to the guidelines that companies must follow to protect the participants in the trial. All of the key facts concerning the trial must be described to the volunteer within informed consent documents. The information will include the following:

- Why the research is being done
- What the researchers wish to accomplish
- What will be done during the trial and the timeline involved
- What risks are involved in the trial
- What benefits can be expected from the trial
- What other treatments are available

These documents should be studied carefully, and any questions should be asked before a decision is made. If a person decides to join a clinical trial, she will be asked to sign a consent form. Under informed consent, participants may ask questions or withdraw at any time before, during, or after the trial.

Fact

Every clinical trial in the United States must be approved and monitored by an Institutional Review Board (IRB) to make sure the risks are as low as possible and are worth any potential benefits. An IRB is an independent committee of physicians, statisticians, community advocates, and others that ensures that a clinical trial is ethical and the rights of study participants are protected.

Should You Participate?

There are a variety of reasons people choose to join a clinical trial. The prospect of receiving a new treatment before it is available to the public is alluring to many people who are excited about a treatment's potential benefit. Contributing to research and society is another reason people want to participate.

In general, people who volunteer for clinical trials report a positive experience. A recent survey found that 54 percent of the people polled rated their experience as excellent. Still, it is important to understand the pros and cons of this volunteer opportunity. Here are some questions you should ask before making a decision:

- Why is the research being done?
- Has the study been reviewed and approved?
- Why does the research team think the experimental medical intervention will work?
- Where will the clinical trial take place?
- How often will I have to go to the study site?
- How long is the clinical trial?
- What type of therapies, tests, and procedures will the participants have?
- Will the therapies, tests, and procedures be painful?
- Will participants have medical care after the study ends? If so, who provides it?
- How will the therapies, tests, and procedures compare to those for the regular treatment?
- Will participants be able to take their regular treatment and drugs during the clinical trial?
- What happens if I am harmed by the experimental medical intervention?

As you can see, there is quite a bit to consider before deciding whether or not to participate in a clinical trial. Here are the pros to consider:

- You may be among the first to benefit from a new treatment.
- You'll be helping others by contributing to medical research.
- You'll be closely monitored and receive high-quality medical care.

Weigh those against the cons:

- Experimental treatments may bring unpleasant or serious side effects.
- The treatment may not work for you, or it may end up being less effective than the available treatment.
- You may receive a placebo.

- Participating may require more of your time and energy than a normal treatment regimen.
- There may be more tests and doctor visits.
- Your health plan may not cover all your costs.
- You may have to change doctors.

Before deciding to participate in a trial, it is imperative that you speak with your MS specialist first. She knows you best and will be able to help you make an informed decision.

Question

Are people paid for their time in clinical trials?
Some, but not all, studies pay their participants. Somewhere between 33 and 40 percent of the 80,000 industry- and publicly funded human studies under way pay their subjects. Each year, 2.5 million people participate in research studies involving human subjects.

Do Your Homework

Staying abreast of new treatments and therapies should be an important part of your management plan. But you'll also want to get a handle on your current medical care. Do your homework! A recent survey revealed that up to 50 percent of Americans at all socioeconomic levels struggle with health literacy, defined as the ability to read, understand, and act on spoken and written health information from medical professionals. And according to the Health Literacy Coalition, 80 percent of patients forget what doctors tell them as soon as they leave the office. This means there are a whole lot of people who are uneducated and confused about their medical conditions!

The complexities of multiple sclerosis make it a rather complicated subject to grasp, and other factors, such as complex medical terms and difficulties in communicating with your doctor, don't make it any easier. People often feel embarrassed to admit that they don't know something and fail to ask for help. Being an informed patient and staying on top of new treatments and developments will give you the edge you need to manage your illness.

Effective Communication

It's important that you shoulder some of the responsibility when speaking to your doctor by taking notes and asking questions, but you also have the right to be spoken to in a language you can understand. This means that your doctor should be willing to skip the medical jargon and speak to you in layman's terms. While the medical community is increasingly requiring patients to take responsibility for their own care, sometimes what is asked of them is beyond their capacity to comprehend. Ask your doctor to use visual aids, such as a picture of the central nervous system, when describing functions or conditions. In general, people seem to remember key points better when a visual aid is used to emphasize a point.

Essential

Some medical offices are beginning to post treatment plans online so patients can log on when needed; if this isn't available, have your doctor write out any information as a backup. It is also important to talk to your doctor about new treatments or information that interests you. Schedule an appointment apart from regular visits to discuss your ideas.

Research

The first thing to do before you begin research on multiple sclerosis is to get organized. Purchase a notebook where you take and keep notes. Here are some other helpful tips for researching your condition:

- **Cast a wide net.** Your doctor isn't the only one who has information on multiple sclerosis, although you should always use him as your primary source. Don't forget that pharmacists, CAM practitioners, medical librarians, and other nonprofessionals may have the information that you're looking for.

- **Surf the Internet.** The Internet is a great place to find education and support, but it's a two-sided coin. A good amount of information that you'll find online is outdated or erroneous. The key is knowing where to look. Once you get the hang of it, you can navigate your way to the websites with the best information. Typically, government and university sites are the best resources, along with organizations and societies dedicated to MS. The pharmaceutical companies that manufacture the MS medications are also a good resource, but keep in mind that those sites also contain marketing messages.

- **Find out about clinical studies.** Clinical studies are a great way to become familiar with new treatments in the pipeline, but they can be somewhat hard to read and interpret. In their basic form, they're divided into several sections, with the abstract (summary of key points), the results (where the data is summarized), and the discussion or conclusion sections the most important from a lay perspective. Significant studies usually make their way into articles, journals, and websites where they've been rewritten for the general public.

- **Visit your library.** If you don't have a medical library nearby (such as a university or hospital library), your public library may have a wealth of information on hand. Ask your librarian to help you find current journal or newspaper articles on MS and browse the catalogue of books pertaining to the subject.

Well-meaning friends and relatives often have a plethora of tips and ideas for the person with MS. If something sounds interesting, do your own research and check with your doctor. A good way to handle unsolicited advice is to thank them for the information and tell them you'll look into it at a later time.

Staying One Step Ahead

So, you're working on your checklist. You've decided on (or have started) a disease-modifying therapy, you've created a health care team, done your research, and created a support network. Now what? Planning for your future is your next most important step. You want to create a life full of hope and determination while keeping an eye on practical matters, such as financial planning, employment issues, and unanticipated surprises.

Dealing with Unpredictability

After hearing from your doctor that you have MS, one of the first pictures to cross your mind may have been a wheelchair. This is an all too common response, owed to various media images that have crossed our paths or because of the misconceptions about MS that exist in the minds of the general public. By now you've come to understand that the majority of people with MS remain mobile throughout their lives and that their life expectancy is on a par with the rest of the general population. And these days, therapies increase the chances that people with MS will live with little disability for longer times.

The reality is, however, that for most people, the DMTs don't completely stop relapses, and despite all of the good news in the MS arena, a percentage of people with MS face some type of disability. While you're sitting tight waiting for a cure, it's important to get a handle on your future. And while you may never need to access any of these safety nets, knowing that you're prepared brings peace of mind. Here are some tips to help you get started:

- Understand the disease course of MS. A percentage of people with relapsing-remitting MS transition to a more progressive course within twenty-five years.
- Anticipate a change in your income. Hope for the best, but plan for the worst. A good financial planner can help you strategize for the future, taking into account your assets, savings, and current expenses.

- Review your insurance plans. This is essential. Know the who, what, where, and why of your health care coverage, life insurance, and disability policies. In other words, read the fine print and ask questions now.
- Keep good records. That means filing all insurance claims, medical records, receipts, and prescriptions and any other paperwork pertaining to your condition.
- Assess your employment status. Your job security needs to be taken into account so you can better plan for the future. Is now the time to switch jobs? Change careers? Go back to school?
- Create a management team that can help you with any future issues, such as social security attorneys, financial planners, career counselors, or social workers.
- Know the laws in your state that apply to employment, health, and disability. The laws are there to protect you.

The field of MS research holds a lot of promise for those who are living with this illness, and for those who will be diagnosed in the years ahead. The past decade has uncovered new clues, diagnostic techniques and treatments—and the next ten years look even more promising. Staying one step ahead by doing your homework, communicating with your health care team, and setting realistic goals for yourself will help you to manage MS until the next generation of therapies—and hopefully a cure—comes to the forefront.

CHAPTER 19

Creating a Support Network

RESEARCH SHOWS THAT healthy relationships can reduce stress and improve your overall health and sense of well-being. Support networks also promote a sense of belonging, boost your self-worth, and underscore your feelings of security. A network can consist of friends, family members, coworkers, or key players on your health care team, but in this chapter, you'll focus on social support—the people in your life who provide emotional sustenance.

Reaching Out

Most people are just plain uncomfortable asking others for assistance. They often feel as if they are conveying an undesirable message about themselves when they admit they need some help. Here are some common myths that need to be debunked:

- **Asking for help makes you look weak or needy.** On the contrary, asking for help is a sign of strength. Recognizing that you are having difficulty managing certain aspects of your life is the first step in finding a solution.

- **Asking for help signals incompetence.** Here's a reality check: no one can do it all. That's why there are tax accountants and plumbers. It's important to let go of your need to be perfect.
- **Asking for help puts others in an awkward position.** Trust other people to know their own limits and to say no when they're not able to assist you.
- **Asking for help might lead to rejection.** It might, but chances are the people in your life will be happy to help. If someone can't be there for you this time, you can cast a wider net and enlist the support of others.

Independence and self-sufficiency are admirable qualities, but the best ventures in life are created by teamwork and mutual support. Reaching out to friends and family strengthens your bonds with them and allows you to feel intimately connected. And don't forget that when people lend support, it makes them feel good about themselves. Providing an opportunity for others to share in your life contributes to their own sense of well-being, too.

Self-esteem can play a role in determining whether or not you reach out for help. You have to feel worthy of another's time and attention. Remember that you deserve a hand as much as anyone else, and once someone answers your mayday call, it will reinforce the message that you're worthy.

Essential

The Chronic Illness Workbook by Patricia Fennell identifies four progressive phases of change in people living with chronic conditions: crisis, stabilization, resolution, and integration. This is an effective book to help people to develop effective management strategies to live their lives to the fullest.

If you've never been inclined to ask for help, it may take some practice. Picture the last time you asked someone for help. Did it feel uncomfortable? Did you apologize three times before hanging up the phone? Many people struggle to enlist the care and support of others.

It's important to be specific about what you need. Since many MS symptoms are invisible, it's not always readily apparent what you may want or need. Don't expect your husband to jump in and get the dishes done when you're dead tired unless he knows the extent of your fatigue. Communicating effectively and being assertive are good ways to let people know how you're doing and what needs to be done. Your best friend doesn't know your bladder is acting up or that you're working through muscle spasms unless you tell her. If you've always folded the laundry, don't expect the kids to jump in unless you've explained to them that Mom's a bit tired today. The truth is, you have to send a clear message by being specific. Never assume that anyone knows what you need or how you're feeling.

Fact

The National Institute of Neurological Disorders and Stroke (NINDS) has a mission to reduce the burden of neurological disease. Their website, *www.ninds.nih.gov*, is a good resource for research and includes information on clinical trials, current news, and a list of organizations pertaining to MS.

Cultivating Your Support Network

The first step toward developing a strong support network is evaluating your own behavior as it relates to building and maintaining relationships. Relationships, after all, are a two-way street. The better friend or relative you are, the better your relationships will be.

Staying in touch by answering phone calls, sending e-mails, and making lunch dates keep you connected to the people in your life. You have to nurture those relationships. Even when you're having a relapse or a particularly bad week, sending a quick e-mail or leaving a voice mail will let others know you are still there and are eager to spend time with them once you're feeling better. Being proactive about your relationships puts part of the responsibility for their maintenance on your own plate: initiate an invitation, make plans for a rainy day.

People like to hear that they're appreciated. Send thank-you notes and express your gratitude. There are a million ways to let them know they're an important part of your life.

 Alert

> Look for ways to manage unhealthy relationships, especially those you can't avoid, such as a nagging in-law. Some evidence shows that the negative consequences of maintaining obligatory relationships, such as with certain relatives or coworkers, can outweigh the benefits. Relationships should add to your sense of well-being rather than adding to your stress levels.

Being in a healthy relationship means you're traveling down a two-way street. Being a good listener is one of the most important aspects of communication. Even though you might cringe when you listen to your Aunt Mary's sixth recital of her bunion operation, perhaps your Aunt Mary was there when you needed someone to pick up the kids from school or she baked all the pies at Thanksgiving. A relationship means that you give and take and you're there for one another when needed. Listening to the woes of others is sometimes part of the package.

Friends as Support

In the spectrum of a year, people grow and change in myriad and unforeseen ways. Your feelings, your interests, and even your ideas move along with the natural ebb and flow of life. Relationships change, too; friends come in and out of your life, their life circumstances as unpredictable and unyielding as yours. It is a gift, then, to harbor those friends who seem to stay with you through it all, whose love and companionship are unconditional and forgiving.

People who have lived through difficult times have no problem identifying those unshakeable friendships. They're the friends who will call in sick to get you to a doctor's appointment, drive through the rain to pass the Kleenex to you, or call to ask you to go fishing when they know you've had a long week.

There are other friends, too, who live in the periphery of your days—maybe a high school friend who doesn't live close but who's always been good for a laugh on the phone. Or there are the friends you see on occasion, such as those who share your interests or hobbies. Different friends serve different needs in your life. It's a good idea to figure out how each person makes up the different pieces of your puzzle.

Because people are all different, their reaction to your diagnosis of MS is likely to be as varied as they are. The Pollyanna of your friends might have tried to cheer you up with a latte and a speech, while your less expressive friend may have downloaded twenty-five articles on MS from the Internet. Some people whom you'd depended upon in the past might have faded from the landscape.

There are many reasons why some people have a hard time dealing with other people's health issues. Some are uncomfortable about their own mortality and don't like to be reminded that bad things happen to good people. Others aren't sure how to respond or how they should help, and so they find it easier to do nothing. And sometimes, a relationship that was based on a shared interest or activity fizzles out if you are no longer able to participate. As sad as this is, it's not uncommon.

Your job, then, is to focus on those relationships that sustain you. And it's equally important to leave yourself open to new friendships. Even with all of your time constraints, MS symptoms, and other obligations, remember that new friendships pop up in the most interesting places—support groups, on the playground, or at work.

It's good to have a toolkit for friendship—a set of guidelines that will help both of you weather the changes that can occur with MS.

Question

Where can mothers with MS find support?
Support groups are a great way to find other women who are living with MS. MS Moms (*www.msmoms.com*) is a website that provides support and advice. In addition, *Women Living with Multiple Sclerosis: Conversations on Living, Loving and Coping* by Judith Nichols is like a portable MS support group for women.

Educate Your Friends

Sharing your knowledge about MS with your friends is important. You may have to cancel an outing from time to time because you're too tired to get off the couch. If your friends understand your symptoms, they'll understand that your life can vary from day to day and they'll be less apt to have misgivings when plans change. Since MS can have an effect on your friendships, you have to give them the tools to adapt. Sharing your knowledge is like lending them a tool.

Look for Changes

If it's been a while since you checked in with an important person in your life, call him and say hello. Although the pace of relationships can change like the tide depending on life circumstances, you can sometimes sense when a friendship has gone astray. Voice your concerns and let your friend know you've got a vested interest in keeping the relationship on track.

You may have to remind yourself that other people have an emotional response to your MS, one that they may be reluctant to discuss with you. But like you, they may be mourning your diagnosis, have fears about your future, and feel saddened by the changes that may or may not occur in your relationship. The diagnosis of a life-changing condition does not happen in a bubble; it's more like a ripple that spreads out from you and affects everyone in your life, including your friends. You might want to encourage your friends to open up about how they're feeling, too.

Be There

If you're having a bad weekend with spasticity and you've been holed up on the couch watching basketball, your best friend may be reluctant to call up and go over the details of his skiing trip. His reluctance is based on concern and respect for you and his intentions are coming from a good place. But the negative consequence to his action, of course, is that you're missing out on a part of his life. Friends like to share the details of their days and you should encourage them to do so. It's no fun to feel as if people are tiptoeing around you, doing their best to avoid hurting your feelings. Friends are there for one another, interested in sharing one another's lives, whether you were there to participate in an event or not. A fair flow of exchange is necessary to strengthen and grow friendships.

Different Folks for Different Strokes

Since you are closer to some friends than you are to others and relationships serve different purposes in your life, some friends will be more responsive to certain needs than others. You probably intuit this and already respect certain boundaries without knowing you're doing it. You know which friend you can call up past 10:00 P.M., which friend is more likely to help you move, and which friend will take your kids for a night. Making these types of distinctions between your support group members is important.

Reciprocate

Healthy relationships are based on mutual need and respect, so the old "do unto others" rule is a good one. There doesn't have to be a scorecard involved or an invisible line drawn in the sand, but no one wants to be on the heavy end of the teeter-totter for long. Give back. And remember that it's the little things you do for others that matter most.

Family as Support

See your support system as a diagram of concentric circles with you as the center. Your family represents the circles closest to you. Of those who surround you in life, MS impacts your family the most; by the same token, they are typically your main source of support. For those with advanced MS, spouses and other family members are sometimes caregivers—those who assist with your daily activities to one degree or another.

No matter what level of support is required at home, it's important to find a balance between supportive activity and relationship. Compromise and flexibility are called upon if a family member can no longer participate in activities you once enjoyed. Finding new ways to do old things is imperative; maintaining familial social ties and contributing to the emotional aspects of relationships are equally important. In other words, you must create a space where MS is minimized or put aside. Sharing news, laughing, bonding through hobbies and interests—these are the spaces where relationships bloom and grow.

Extended family—grandparents, cousins, and uncles—may also play a big role in your support network, especially those who live close to you. Tell them you'll let them know when you need them, and then let them know what you need. Make sure you're not counting on one or two people to provide support. That can be hard on them and hard on you if they're not there when you need them. Beyond family, you should cultivate relationships with friends, support group members, and mentors that inspire you. Variety is the key.

Support Groups

Finding people who share common ground can bring a great sense of comfort and relief. Talking to someone else who knows exactly what you mean when you describe tingling hands, electric-shock sensations, or blurry vision can be life-affirming. You can describe what you're feeling to friends and family, but to actually talk to someone who knows it from experience is a different story.

Support groups can take several forms, from an intimate gathering of several people who have MS to organized groups that meet in hospitals or churches. The Internet is also another way to connect with people who are living with MS. Whatever type of gathering you choose, you are bound to find camaraderie and learn a great deal in the process. You might be interested in seeing how others are coping with the disease, or you can just share tips and find occasional humor in the shared trials of living with MS.

Essential

There are more than 1,000 support groups listed on the *www.selfhelpgroups.org* website, so if you're looking for an online support network, this may be a good place to start. In addition, *www.mentalhelp.net/selfhelp* has a searchable database to help you find organizations and groups by typing in a keyword.

Support group gatherings can be eye-openers to newly diagnosed folks, as you're likely to meet others living with various types of MS and in all different stages. If you're just sticking your toe in the water, you may want to find a newly diagnosed group, as the topics of conversation may be more geared to the sorts of things you're experiencing: medical tests, diagnostic issues, and similar symptoms. But there's something to be said about meeting those people who have years of experience managing their MS; they've got plenty of wisdom and knowledge to share.

Most organized groups have a facilitator who runs the meetings. Guest speakers such as neurologists, urologists, financial planners, and other professionals are often invited to speak and answer questions.

If your community offers choices, it may take you a while to find a group that suits you. Some areas have specific groups, such as gay and lesbian support groups, groups for the newly diagnosed, or groups for advanced MS. You might find that one group spends too much time on complaining, or another is too chatty about personal matters, but generally, organized groups are focused on support and education.

The best way to find out what's available is by asking your doctor or calling your local chapter of the NMSS, which you can find on the NMSS website (*www.nationalmssociety.org*) or by calling 1-800-FIGHT-MS. The NMSS offers programs, lectures, and conferences that provide another way to meet and network with others. Getting involved is a good way to develop new friendships and stay on top of the latest news and treatments.

Internet Support

The Internet provides a great service to those living with MS by promoting a sense of community and by granting instant access to educational tools. People with mobility issues, especially, enjoy a sense of ease and convenience by turning on their computers and finding support. There's also comfort in anonymity for some. Interestingly, you'll find the same sort of group dynamics you witness in any organization where competition and in-house bickering pop up from time to time. But Internet groups provide the same "I've been there" support and, unlike anything in this world, offer people the ability to connect with one another and experience what is, in essence, instant group therapy. Here's a rundown on some of the sites you can visit to find support:

- The National Multiple Sclerosis Society (NMSS) funds research and provides more services, support, and information than any other MS organization. They also advocate on behalf of people with MS at the local and national level. Their website is full of educational opportunities, including webcasts, online pamphlets, and current news and trends in treatment and research. They can also refer you to specialists in your area, including neurologists, mental health professionals, and other supporting players in MS-related issues. Their website (*www.nationalmssociety.org*) can also help you locate a support group or local chapter of the NMSS in your area.

- The Multiple Sclerosis Foundation (MSF) is another nonprofit organization providing support and services to people with MS. Along with educational programs and regional support groups, they boast a lending library from which people with MS can borrow books that are shipped to them by mail. Their website (*www.msfocus.org*) includes news articles, a moderated chat room, and information on ordering free MSF publications, including brochures, fact sheets, a newsletter, and a lifestyle magazine.
- MSWorld (*www.msworld.org*) connects individuals with MS to a variety of chat rooms and message boards and boasts a "patients helping patients" theme. A lively monthly column, book reviews, special guest chats, and links to resources make this a popular website.
- The Multiple Sclerosis International Federation (*www.msif. org*) links more than eighty MS organizations worldwide and has forty-three member societies. Their website boasts resource and research pages and connects visitors to regional support groups.
- Multiple Sclerosis Association of America (MSAA) is a national nonprofit organization that provides support and direct services to people with MS. Their website provides a list of their services and educational opportunities offered throughout the country. Their website is *www.msaa.org*.

If you are isolated—live far away from your extended family or have recently moved to a new area—it's important to be proactive about expanding your social support network. Studies show that having one or two close and supportive friends is at least as valuable to emotional health as having a large group of friendly acquaintances, so it's not the quantity that counts, but the quality. Joining a gym, volunteering, and developing new interests and hobbies can provide you with opportunities to seek out and establish relationships with others.

CHAPTER 20

Advanced MS and the Caregiver's Role

A SMALL PERCENTAGE of people with MS will progress to a more advanced stage that may require skilled care. Although relatively few families will confront the issues of advanced MS, the following chapter is directed to those who do. It's likely that at this point in time, your family and friends have been living with your MS for a long time and have adapted gradually as you've bravely weathered the changes over the years. The second half of this chapter is devoted to the people who care for you and is full of tips and resources to help them with the day-to-day issues of caregiving.

Treatment for Advanced MS

You may have had a progressive form of MS right from the start, or perhaps you were initially diagnosed with a relapsing-remitting course that has become steadily progressive. In either case, there are few treatment options available right now for progressive forms of MS. And while that is discouraging, some of the drugs in the pipeline look promising. In the meantime, though, your neurologist is likely to have a few tricks up his sleeve, and with effective symptom management and support, you can maintain a high quality of life.

The six disease-modifying drugs available for MS target those who experience relapses, including relapsing-remitting, and some types of secondary progressive MS. Those with primary progressive MS and secondary progressive MS without relapses may not be appropriate candidates for these therapies. The good news is that your doctor may recommend some other options including the following.

Novantrone (mitoxantrone)

This chemotherapy drug is often prescribed for folks with secondary progressive MS, with or without relapses. It has a lifetime dose limit because of heart complications, but it's been shown to slow down or reduce the progression of disability in some patients. Novantrone is not FDA-approved for people with primary progressive MS.

Question

Do more men or women get PPMS?
Twice as many women are diagnosed with RRMS than men, whereas PPMS is divided equally between the sexes. Some sources report a slight tendency toward more men than women being diagnosed with this form of MS. The onset of PPMS is generally after age thirty-five, with many people being diagnosed in their forties or fifties.

Immunosuppressants

Immunosuppressants have been used to suppress the immune system in people with MS who are not experiencing relapses. Chemotherapy drugs such as Imuran (azathioprine), Cytoxan (cyclophosphamide), and methotrexate can be used and seem to be effective in altering the course of the disease for some people.

Treatments on the Horizon

Researchers around the world are striving to discover better diagnostic criteria and possible treatment options for progressive MS. Research may unveil a line of MS drugs and therapies that repair and regenerate lost myelin and nerve fibers (axons). The drugs may have the potential to restore function, which is an important goal in MS research. Some agents are showing this type of action in animal studies, but the transition from animal studies to human trials can be lengthy and difficult.

Neuroprotection is another area of interest for the treatment of all types of MS. This type of treatment would potentially protect the central nervous system from damage caused by an attack from the body's immune-system cells. The hope is that nerves and myelin would remain more intact, and patients would have fewer symptoms.

Researchers hope it will be just a matter of time before individuals with PPMS have access to new disease-modifying therapies.

Tips on Managing Advanced MS

Managing your MS means taking care of all of you—your physical and emotional well-being. You goal is to function at an optimal level, despite all of the challenges you may face. You'll want to lean on your management team and support network to keep you happy and comfortable, with an eye toward your valued independence.

Symptom Management

Managing the symptoms of progressive MS will take the skill and know-how of your management team. As you learned in Chapter 9, symptoms can be effectively managed and so your job is to be proactive and stay one step ahead of them. The goal of symptom management is to find relief and to keep you as comfortable as possible, so be the squeaky wheel at your doctor's office. There are three types of symptoms you should monitor:

- *Primary symptoms* are directly caused by MS and can include weakness, balance problems, bowel and bladder problems, and vision impairment.
- *Secondary symptoms* are complications that arise from primary symptoms. For example, bladder symptoms can give way to urinary tract infections; skin problems can arise from lack of mobility; and fatigue can result from certain medications.
- *Tertiary symptoms* include the psychological and social effects of living with MS. Transferring certain aspects of self-care to others can cause problems with self-esteem and lead to depression. Certain symptoms may cause you to withdraw from others or limit enjoyable activities.

It's important to stay on top of all three types of symptoms, as treatment can vastly improve the quality of your life.

Fact

It has long been assumed that people with PPMS have less inflammatory damage to the CNS than those with RRMS. But recent studies indicate that there may be significant inflammation in the CNS in people with PPMS. These findings may point to better evaluation of disease activity in PPMS and may open the door for this patient population to be included in therapeutic trials.

Staying Healthy

You may be skeptical, but even those with mobility and weakness issues can find a way to stretch their muscles and exercise their bodies. Your rehabilitation team will be an invaluable tool in this pursuit. You also want to be sure you have yearly physicals and keep a good eye on your general health.

Alert

If you're doing all of your workouts at home, you might want to think about investing in some specialized exercise equipment. There are many new strength-training machines available for people with disabilities, as well as hand-cyclers and other cardio equipment. Check out *www. disabilityonline.com.*

Occupational Therapy

Occupational therapists can help you get on with the tasks of day-to-day living. They are armed with solutions and advice to help you perform activities such as bathing, dressing, and cooking. An occupational therapist will assess your living environment to see whether you need assistive devices and can also recommend strengthening and stretching exercises, especially for the arms, to your physical therapist that may be beneficial for you.

Other Rehabilitation Specialists

Rehabilitation—including physical therapy, speech therapy, and cognitive retraining—can help you manage—even reduce—certain cognitive and physical challenges. Here are some of the players on your rehab team:

- **Physical therapist.** Your physical therapist can help you in your ability to perform daily tasks and may even help you feel better.
- **Speech therapist.** Speech therapists may improve your communication skills if you have speech difficulties. They can also help you with swallowing problems.

- **Cognitive rehabilitation.** Cognitive retraining can help you manage problems with thinking, reasoning, and remembering. Your neurologist can recommend a neuropsychologist to you.

Rehabilitation may help you live a more productive life, especially if your symptoms are constant or severe. One of the primary goals of rehabilitation is to help prevent physical complications that may occur with MS. Your doctor can help you figure out which types of rehabilitation will be most beneficial to you. Rehabilitation can take place on an outpatient basis or for inpatients in a rehabilitation center.

Mental Health Issues

You'll want to keep an eye out for depression and address any issues that are having a negative impact on your emotional health. Mental health professionals can help you identify areas in your life that need work, including self-esteem issues, lack of resources and social support, and depression. Here are some of the people you can call on for help:

- **Social worker.** A social worker can hook you up with all sorts of local resources such as housing and estate planning. Some social workers also do psychotherapy.
- **Psychotherapist.** In addition to social workers, clinical psychologists and psychiatrists provide psychotherapy. This therapy can help you develop problem-solving skills, deal with the demands of managing an illness, and help you get a grip on the relationships in your life.

The most important word to remember is *proactive*. Always insist that there is more that can be done to help you manage your symptoms. You'll want to make sure the professionals on your management team feel the same way. It is equally important to be proactive about that status of your mental health.

Spiritual Support

Don't underestimate your spiritual needs. Finding a way to cope with the challenges of MS can be a difficult process. Framing your journey within the context of spirituality adds another dimension of support. Talk to a pastor, priest, or rabbi. There are also spiritual counselors who are nondenominational.

Assistive Technology

Members of your rehab team can help you identify adaptive devices that can greatly improve quality of life issues. Whether it's a scooter to get you back on track with your afternoon excursions outdoors or a cane to make walking through the mall a little easier, it's good to have a variety of devices so you don't limit your choice of activities. You want to develop a "can-do" attitude, so figure out what you want to do and can do—and then make it happen. Adaptive sports have come a long way in the past twenty years and now include adaptive skiing, kayaking, canoeing, and even water-skiing, among other activities. Travel for people with disabilities has also exploded, and there are more opportunities than ever before to see the world with assistive technology as one of your companions. Assistive devices can also help people with educational and employment issues.

Options for Care

Families coping with the physical and mental challenges of advanced MS have different options to consider if they decide outside help is needed. They range from adult day care services to opportunities for assisted living. Planning who will provide assistance and care involves several important considerations.

This isn't a topic anyone wants to broach before it is necessary, but it's always a good idea to understand the types of assistance that are available well before they're needed. Look at this as Plan B—another issue you're willing to look into while remaining optimistic.

Determine Needs

Needs are apt to change over time, so decisions related to the best care for you or your loved one will be made more easily if planning has been started early. Your needs will determine the types of resources you seek out. Draft a plan that considers the best care options, updating it over time as needs and resources change. List the sorts of care that may be needed, such as help with hygiene, transportation, and assistive devices. Seek out a social worker who can help you locate community-based resources and programs.

Insurance Issues

Your first concern should be health care—especially insurance coverage. Take a look at what kind of insurance coverage you have and discuss any changes that might be prudent. Educate yourself about Medicaid, Medicare, Medigap, and long-term care insurance. Check your insurance plan for details on home health care, assisted living, and nursing home coverage. Since policies differ greatly in coverage, it's important to assess your financial obligations when making choices.

Home Care Options

Even if you need frequent nursing care, you can remain at home and arrange for in-home nursing care and housekeeping services. Depending on the area you live in, there are a variety of resources to consider:

- **Adult day programs.** Adult day programs are planned programs of weekday activities designed to promote well-being through social and health-related services. Care centers can be public or private, nonprofit or for-profit.
- **Meals and transportation.** Most communities offer programs to assist with meals or transportation, such as Meals on Wheels and programs that utilize accessible buses and vans.
- **Home care services.** Trained personnel can help manage the day-to-day basics at home, such as bathing, meal preparation,

and medical and therapeutic routines. These programs are usually privately paid.

- **Respite care.** These programs bring a trained person into the home for short visits so that caregivers can take time off to do the shopping, go to medical appointments, or take time out for themselves. There may be some state or federal funding available for these services.

Long-Term Care

Long-term care is designed to meet the physical, social and emotional needs of people who require twenty-four-hour care and supervision.

- **Assisted living.** Assisted living is for adults who need help with everyday tasks but don't need full-time nursing care. Some assisted-living facilities are part of retirement communities.
- **Nursing home care.** This option provides twenty-four-hour care by skilled staff members and is often used when other caregiving options have been ruled out or exhausted. While this is certainly a difficult decision, sometimes nursing homes are the best place for people who need nursing and personal care. There are a variety of homes to choose from, ranging from homelike to hospital-like. There are some good books and websites to help you explore this option as there is a great deal to consider and research. It's a good idea to inquire about the history of the nursing or other care homes that you're interested in by visiting state regulatory agencies or by visiting *www.medicare.gov.*

As with any important endeavor, it's always a good idea to talk with friends, neighbors, and your local area agency on aging or health to learn more about the home health care agencies in your community.

The Caregiver's Role

Whether you moved into the role of caregiver fairly quickly or gradually over time, you are likely to have questions and concerns about your role. You've probably learned a great deal on your own and have become adept at matching resources with your loved one's needs.

You may have already sensed how important it is to take care of yourself, too. Through this book, you've learned how important it is for all people to take responsibility for their own health and happiness, even when it may be hard to do so.

Each caregiver defines his role differently, but all caregivers have certain needs of their own that must be met. It may be useful to break these needs into four categories:

- **Help with decision-making.** Having access to educational tools and a strong support network can help you make better decisions, whether they're legal, medical, or financial. Your main goal is to get the needs of your loved one met and then take care of yourself.
- **Need for ease.** You lead a busy life, so find a way to simplify and prioritize. Be on the lookout for products or services that allow you to complete tasks quickly. Whenever possible, get help with household tasks by hiring someone else to do them for you.
- **Peace of mind.** Once the needs of your loved one are met and you've handled the tasks of caregiving, you can shift your focus to other things, such as the needs of other family members or work. Sometimes peace of mind comes from finding other options for care, such as home health care or respite programs.
- **Time for yourself.** This is an easy thing to neglect but vital to your well-being. Time alone can mean an afternoon at the movies or a week at the beach. Finding solutions that allow for personal time and pampering result in healthier, more emotionally stable care providers.

If you are caring for a loved one at home, you are not alone. According to the National Family Caregivers Association, family caregiving is the United State's bedrock when it comes to health care. The services provided by family caregivers represent 80 percent of all home care services and are conservatively valued at $257 billion a year, more than twice the amount spent on paid home care and nursing home services combined.

Tips for Caregivers

Caring for someone you love can be a rewarding experience, but you'll want to watch out for your own emotional health. Caregivers are prone to the experience of "caregiver burnout," which is a state of physical, emotional, and mental exhaustion that may be accompanied by a change in attitude. If you're not getting the help you need, or you're trying to do too much, you may exposing yourself to burnout. Caregivers who are burned out may experience fatigue, stress, anxiety, and depression. Many caregivers also feel guilty if they spend time on themselves.

Fact

More than 50 million people provide care for a chronically ill, disabled, or aged family member or friend during any given year. The typical family caregiver is a forty-six-year-old woman caring for her widowed mother who does not live with her. She is married and employed. Approximately 60 percent of family caregivers are women.

Check out caregiving support groups in your area or talk to a therapist. It's important to find someone you trust so you can express your feelings and frustrations. Support groups allow you to meet others in situations much like yours. You can talk, vent, and exchange tips and hints with people who understand. For those who cannot easily leave home, check out online message boards and forums. It's also good to have a strong support network including professionals, friends, neighbors, and coworkers.

It's essential to be realistic. You can't do everything. Even hospitals and nursing homes rely on a team approach to function, and you should do the same. Turn to other family members for support and to help with tasks.

Taking care of yourself is not a luxury; it's a necessity. Setting aside time each day to read a book or take a nap is a good way to rejuvenate. Take advantage of respite services, which provide a temporary break for caregivers

Alert

A study in the *Journal of the American Medical Association* has shown that those providing care for a spouse become sick more often and experience more stress than people who aren't caregivers. Make sure that you get regular medical checkups. If you have any symptoms of depression, see a doctor right away. Depression is an illness that can, and should, be treated.

Make a list of jobs you need help with and seek out someone to assist you. This could include household chores, running errands, driving, or finding information on services you need.

Caregiving is an act of love, but it can also be a demanding and challenging job. No one can handle it alone. Getting help for yourself is one of the best things you can do—not just for yourself but for your loved one, too. It will enable you to keep giving the best care possible.

Additional Resources

Books

Blackstone, Margaret. *The First Year: Multiple Sclerosis: An Essential Guide for the Newly Diagnosed.* (New York: Marlowe & Company, 2002)

Bowling, Allen C. *Complementary and Alternative Medicine and Multiple Sclerosis.* (New York: Demos Medical Publishing, 2007)

Bowling A. C. and T. M. Stewart. *Dietary Supplements and Multiple Sclerosis: A Health Professional's Guide.* (New York: Demos Medical Publishing, 2004)

Cousins, Norman. *Anatomy of an Illness as Perceived by the Patient.* (New York: Bantam, 2005)

Davis, Amelia. *My Story: A Photographic Essay on Life with Multiple Sclerosis.* (New York: Demos Medical Publishing, 2004)

Fishman, Loren M. M.D. and Eric Small. *Yoga and Multiple Sclerosis: A Journey to Health and Healing.* (New York: Demos Medical Publishing, 2007)

Fortgang, Laura Berman. *Living Your Best Life.* (New York: Tarcher/Putnam, 2001)

Gingold, Jeffrey. *Facing the Cognitive Challenges of MS.* (New York: Demos Medical Publishing, 2006)

Hamler, Brad. *Exercises for People with Multiple Sclerosis: A Safe and Effective Program to Fight Fatigue, Build Strength, and Improve Balance.* (Long Island City, NY: Hatherleigh Press, 2006)

Hill, Beth Ann. *Multiple Sclerosis Q & A: Researching Answers to Frequently Asked Questions.* (Devon, UK: Avery Press, 2003)

Kalb, Rosalind, Ph.D., et al. *Multiple Sclerosis for Dummies.* (Hoboken, NJ: Wiley Publishing, 2007)

Kalb, Rosalind, Ph.D. *Multiple Sclerosis: A Guide for Families.* (New York: Demos Medical Publishing, 2006)

Kalb, Rosalind, Ph D. *Multiple Sclerosis: The Questions You Have—The Answers You Need.* (New York: Demos Medical Publishing, 2007)

Kramer, Dean. *Life on Cripple Creek: Essays on Living with Multiple Sclerosis.* (New York: Demos Medical Publishing, 2003)

LaRocca, Nicholas, Ph.D. and Rosalind Kalb, Ph.D. *Multiple Sclerosis: Understanding the Cognitive Challenges.* (New York: Demos Medical Publishing, 2006)

Meyer, Maria M. and Paula Derr. *The Comfort of Home: A Step-by-Step Guide for Multiple Sclerosis Caregivers.* (New York: Demos Medical Publishing, 2006)

Polman, Chris, M.D. et al. *Multiple Sclerosis: The Guide to Treatment and Management.* (New York: Demos Medical Publishing, 2006)

Reeve, Christopher. *Nothing Is Impossible: Reflections on a New Life.* (New York: Ballantine, 2004)

Rogers, Judith. *The Disabled Woman's Guide to Pregnancy and Childbirth.* (New York: Demos Medical Publishing, 2005)

Russell, Margot. *When the Road Turns: Inspirational Stories by and about People with MS.* (Deerfield Beach, FL, 2001)

Schapiro, Randall. *Managing the Symptoms of Multiple Sclerosis.* (New York: Demos Medical Publishing, 2005)

Schwartz, Shelley Peterman. *Multiple Sclerosis: 300 Tips for Making Life Easier.* (New York: Demos Medical Publishing, 2006)

Weil, Andrew and Rosie Daley. *The Healthy Kitchen: Recipes for a Better Body, Life, and Spirit.* (New York: Knopf, 2002)

Internet Resources
National Multiple Sclerosis Society (NMSS)

A website conducted by the NMSS containing extensive information on multiple sclerosis, including treatment options, current research, support groups, and local chapters of the MS Society.

www.nationalmssociety.org

Multiple Sclerosis Foundation (MSF)

The MSF is a service-based nonprofit organization with a mission to ensure the best quality of life for those living with MS. They offer a lending library, comprehensive support, and educational programs.

www.msfacts.org

Multiple Sclerosis Association of America (MSAA)

The MSAA is a national nonprofit organization offering services and programs that enrich the quality of life for those affected by multiple sclerosis. MSAA provides support and direct services to individuals with MS.

www.msassociation.org

Rocky Mountain MS Center: Alternative Medicine Website

This website offers detailed information about many MS-relevant unconventional therapies, including more than 100 different dietary supplements. It also has detailed surveys and a forum.

www.mscenter.org

MS World

This website offers support and information for people living with MS, including chat rooms, a message board, a resource center, and an online magazine.

www.msworld.org

Consortium of Multiple Sclerosis Centers (CMSC)

The CMSC provides information and support to health care professionals specializing in the care of MS. Their website provides information to MS patients.

www.mscare.org

American Autoimmune Related Diseases Association (AARDA)

The AARDA dedicates itself to the eradication of autoimmune diseases. Their website offers patient information on MS.

www.aarda.org

UnderstandingMS.com

UnderstandingMS.com delivers current information on multiple sclerosis, with a focus on treatment and quality of life decisions.

www.understandingms.com

Multiple Sclerosis International Federation (MSIF)

The MSIF links the activities of national MS societies around the world through research, advocacy, and information dissemination. Their website provides research and resources to people with MS.

www.msif.org

Access-Able Travel Source

Their website provides an extensive list of travel agents and tour operators that are experienced in trip planning for travelers with disabilities.

www.access-able.com

Wilderness Inquiry

The Wilderness Inquiry website provides information on wilderness trips for people with disabilities, including individuals with MS.

www.wildernessinquiry.org

Society for the Advancement of Travel for the Handicapped (SATH]

The SATH website provides and promotes accessible tourism information for disabled travelers.

www.sath.org

MSActive Source

The Active Source website offers free consultation to members regarding reimbursement issues for insurance claims. General information about MS is also offered.

www.msactivesource.com

NeedyMeds

The NeedyMeds website offers information on drug company programs to help people gain access to medications that they could otherwise not afford.

www.needymeds.com

Glossary

Alternative medicine

Unconventional treatments used instead of conventional medicine.

Ataxia

The inability to coordinate voluntary muscular movements.

Autoimmune disease

A condition that occurs when the immune system mistakenly attacks and destroys healthy body tissue. MS is thought to be an autoimmune disease.

Avonex

Brand name for interferon beta-1a. One of the disease-modifying MS therapies.

Axon

The nerve fibers that carry messages and information throughout the central nervous system. Axons are often damaged by demyelination.

Benign MS

A form of relapsing-remitting multiple sclerosis used to describe the disease in people who have had MS for fifteen or more years without serious or enduring disability. Benign MS is thought to account for about 5 percent of RRMS.

Betaseron

Brand name for interferon beta-1b. One of the disease-modifying MS therapies.

Biofeedback

A form of unconventional therapy that trains the mind to control physical responses as measured on special instruments.

Blood-brain barrier (BBB)

A structure that alters the permeability of brain capillaries, so that some substances, such as certain drugs, are prevented from entering brain tissue, while other substances are allowed to enter freely.

Central nervous system (CNS)

The largest part of the nervous system, consisting of the brain, optic nerves, and spinal cord.

Cerebrospinal fluid (CSF)

A protective fluid that circulates and maintains pressure around the brain and spinal cord of the central nervous system.

Clinical trials

Research done in human volunteers to determine the efficacy of medications, surgeries, devices, or procedures.

Complementary medicine

An unconventional treatment that is used along with conventional medicine.

Copaxone

Brand name for glatiramer acetate, or copolymer-1. One of the disease-modifying MS therapies.

Cytokine

A class of immunoregulatory molecules that are secreted by cells of the immune system.

Demyelination

A degenerative process that erodes away the myelin sheath that normally protects nerve fibers. Demyelination exposes these fibers and appears to cause problems in nerve impulse conduction that may affect many physical systems.

Estriol

A major pregnancy-related hormone.

Exacerbation

The appearance of new MS symptoms or, less commonly, the worsening of old ones. An exacerbation lasts at least twenty-four hours and is separated from a previous exacerbation by at least one month. Also known as an attack, flare, or relapse.

Experimental allergic encephalomyelitis (EAE)

An autoimmune disease similar to multiple sclerosis that can be induced in animals for research purposes.

Gadolinium

A paramagnetic metal ion. Gadolinium is approved for use with MRI as a contrast agent to provide a clearer picture of body organs and tissues.

Gene

Unit of DNA responsible primarily for the synthesis of proteins.

Herb

Plants or parts of plants that are used for their flavor, aromatic, and medical purposes.

Inflammation

A basic way the body reacts to infection, irritation, or other injury characterized by by redness, pain, swelling, or loss of function.

Interferon

A group of proteins involved in regulating the immune system.

Lupus

An autoimmune disorder that may mimic MS and is characterized by multiple symptoms, including, rash, fatigue, and painful joints.

Lyme disease

A bacterial disease transmitted by ticks that can cause symptoms that resemble MS.

Magnetic resonance imaging (MRI)

A procedure in which a powerful magnet is used to create detailed pictures of areas inside the body. MRI is an important test for diagnosing MS.

McDonald criteria

The newest diagnostic criteria for different types of MS.

Mitoxantrone

An anticancer agent that has immunosuppressant capability.

MS attack

An exacerbation or increase in MS symptoms.

MS lesion

An abnormal change in structure of the brain or spinal cord that is due to injury or disease; also known as an MS plaque.

MS plaque

A lesion in the brain that is characteristic of MS.

Myelin

A white fatty substance that forms an insulating sheath around the nerve fibers (axons).

Nerve impulse

The electronic signal transmitted along the fibers of nerve cells.

Neurologist

A medical doctor who specializes in diagnosing, treating, and managing disorders of the nervous system.

Neuron

A type of cell in the nervous system that can send and receive nerve impulses.

Novantrone

Brand name of mitoxantrone, an anticancer drug that is used to suppress immune cells.

Occupational therapist (OT)

A health care professional who helps patients improve performance in their daily living and working environments.

Optic neuritis

Inflammation of the optic nerve.

Paraparesis

Partial paralysis affecting both legs.

Peripheral nervous system

A network of nerve fibers that transmits information to, and receives information from, the central nervous system.

Placebo

An inactive substance used in controlled experiments testing the effectiveness of an experimental therapy.

Prevalence

The percentage of a population with a particular disease at any given time.

Primary progressive MS (PPMS)

A subtype of MS characterized by slow worsening of symptoms with no perceivable attacks.

Progressive-relapsing MS

A subtype of MS characterized by slow worsening of symptoms from the onset and attacks that begin after the onset of progression.

Rebif

Brand name of interferon beta-1a. One of the disease-modifying MS therapies.

Relapsing-remitting MS

A subtype of MS characterized by distinct exacerbations separated by periods of full or partial recovery.

Secondary progressive MS

A subtype of MS characterized initially by intermittent attacks and subsequently by slowly progressive worsening.

Spasticity

A condition characterized by muscular contraction with increased reflexes.

Statins

A group of drugs that decrease the synthesis of cholesterol and have anti-inflammatory effects.

Stem cell

An unspecialized cell that may develop into one of many different types of specific cells.

Steroid

Natural or synthetic compounds used to treat MS relapses or attacks.

T cell

A type of cell belonging to a class of immune cells known as lympho-cytes. T cells play a central role in a process known as cell-mediated immunity.

Tremor

A trembling or shaking.

Tysabri

An antibody therapy that is effective for treating relapsing-remitting MS.

Vaccination

The administration of material to produce immunity to an infection.

Virus

A large group of noncellular infective agents that can cause disease.

Vitamin

A nutrient compound that is required in tiny amounts by an organism.

Index

The Everything® Health Guide Series

Supportive advice. Real answers.

The Everything® Health Guide to Addiction and Recovery
$14.95, ISBN 10: 1-59869-806-0, ISBN 13: 978-1-59869-806-0

The Everything® Health Guide to Adult Bipolar Disorder
$14.95, ISBN 10: 1-59337-585-9, ISBN 13: 978-1-59337-585-0

The Everything® Health Guide to Arthritis
$14.95, ISBN 10: 1-59869-410-3, ISBN 13: 978-1-59869-410-9

The Everything® Health Guide to Controlling Anxiety
$14.95, ISBN 10: 1-59337-429-1, ISBN 13: 978-1-59337-429-7

The Everything® Health Guide to Depression
$14.95, ISBN 10: 1-59869-407-3 ISBN 13: 978-1-59869-407-9

The Everything® Health Guide to Diabetes
$14.95, ISBN 10: 1-59869-785-4, ISBN 13: 978-1-59869-785-8

The Everything® Health Guide to Fibromyalgia
$14.95, ISBN 10: 1-59337-586-7, ISBN 13: 978-1-59337-586-7

The Everything® Health Guide to Menopause, 2nd Edition
$14.95, ISBN 10: 1-59869-405-7, ISBN 13: 978-1-59869-405-5

The Everything® Health Guide to Multiple Sclerosis
$14.95, ISBN 10: 1-59869-805-2, ISBN 13: 978-1-59869-805-3

The Everything® Health Guide to Migraines
$14.95, ISBN 10: 1-59869-411-1, ISBN 13: 978-1-59869-411-6

The Everything® Health Guide to OCD
$14.95, ISBN 10: 1-59869-435-9, ISBN 13: 978-1-59869-435-2

The Everything® Health Guide to PMS
$14.95, ISBN 10: 1-59869-395-6 ISBN 13: 978-1-59869-395-9

The Everything® Health Guide to Postpartum Care
$14.95, ISBN 10: 1-59869-275-5, ISBN 13: 978-1-59869-275-4

The Everything® Health Guide to Thyroid Disease
$14.95, ISBN 10: 1-59337-719-3, ISBN 13: 978-1-59337-719-9